Seasonal Vegan Macrobiotic Cuisine

ERIC LECHASSEUR & SANAE SUZUKI

love, eric & sanae

Love, Eric & Sanae.
Copyright © 2007 Eric Lechasseur and
Sanae Suzuki.

All rights reserved. Printed in Hong Kong.
No part of this book may be used or reproduced
in any manner whatsoever without written
permission except in the case of brief quotations
embodied in critical articles or reviews.
For information contact mugen, LLC
2610A 23rd Street, Santa Monica, CA 90405.

FIRST EDITION.

www.LoveEricInc.com

ISBN 0-9772937-1-8

Printed with soy-based inks.

Book design by Ellison / Goodreau, Los Angeles.
Introductory text edited by Douglas Clayton.
Recipes edited by X-tine Goodreau.

All photographs by Yoshi Ueda, except pages 19,
33, 53, and 81 by Eric Lechasseur, and pages 37
and 49 by Sanae Suzuki.
Food styling by Sanae Suzuki and Eric Lechasseur.

The ceramic dishes used in the following
photographs were handmade by:
Yoriko Ikuzawa, pages 14, 16, 24, 28, 38, 44, 54,
   56, 60, 62, 66, 70, 72, 82
Eric Lechasseur, pages 20, 50
Michael Marcus, page 72
Michiko Nakamura, pages 24, 34, 40, 70, 72, 82, 86
Sanae Suzuki, pages 16, 46, 50, 88
Yoshihiko Yoshida, page 66
Vladimira Zboril, pages 22, 30, 46

Disclaimer:
The recipes contained in this book should not be used as, or in place of, standard
medical treatment for any sickness or injury of any sort. Individuals deciding on
their dietary choices are responsible for their own health and should consult their
doctor as well as a professional macrobiotic counselor before undertaking any
unusual dietary changes.

For people who are seeking a true macrobiotic way of living that is invigorating, nurturing, and entertaining, while receiving the benefits of the changing seasons.

CONTENTS

- 6   Acknowledgements
- 7   Foreword
- 9   A Note from Eric & Sanae

Spring
- 15   Carrot and Garbanzo Soup with Lotus Root and Dill
- 15   Kombu Dashi
- 17   Leek and Cauliflower Filo Wrap with Mint Sauce
- 18   Country Whole Barley with Fava Beans
- 18   Pressed Wakame and Napa Cabbage Rolls
- 21   Tempeh Crab Cakes with Caper Sauce
- 21   Sautéed Pea Sprouts
- 23   Strawberry Cupcakes
- 25   Apricot Linzer
- 25   Green Tea with Chamomile

Summer Brunch
- 29   Honeydew Melon Soup
- 31   Vegetable Pancakes with Tofu Sour Cream
- 32   Inca Quinoa and Mustard Greens Salad
- 32   Zucchini Muffins
- 35   Scrambled Tofu Florentine with Hollandaise Sauce
- 36   Dulse and Cucumber with Basil
- 39   Grilled Nectarines with Lemon and Maple Glaze
- 41   Hazelnut Baci
- 41   Cool Roasted Corn Tea

Late Summer
- 45   Sweet Corn Chowder with Basil Oil
- 47   Kamut Spaghetti with Pine Nuts and Sun Dried Tomatoes
- 47   Simmered Turnips
- 48   Arame Poppyseed Rolls
- 51   Stuffed Shiitake Mushrooms with Millet and Kudzu Beet Sauce
- 52   Melon and Thai Basil Pickles with Lemongrass
- 55   Pistachio Chocolate Mousse
- 57   Mini Blueberry Scones
- 57   Kukicha with Rose Hips and Petals

Autumn
- 61   Butternut Squash and Kidney Bean Potage
- 63   Root Vegetable Pot Pie
- 64   Breaded Rice Balls with Lotus Seeds
- 65   Shredded Daikon Salad with Pink Peppercorns
- 67   Mihama Hijiki with Edamame and Roasted Pumpkin Seeds
- 67   Lotus Root Pickles
- 68   Persimmon and Watercress with Asian Pear
- 71   Black Sesame Dumplings with Warm Coconut Soup
- 73   Walnut Cookies
- 73   Genmaicha

Winter
- 77   French Onion Soup with Crispy Mochi
- 79   Seitan Bourguignon
- 79   Buckwheat and Brown Rice
- 80   Red Radish and Green Top Pickles
- 80   Crispy Kombu Chips
- 83   Savoy Cabbage with Walnut and Carrot Sauce
- 84   Braised Whole Burdock
- 87   Apple Cinnamon Strudel
- 89   Oatmeal Cherry Kisses
- 89   Soy Latte Grain Coffee

- 90   Basic Essentials Metric Conversions
- 91   Index
- 98   Glossary

ACKNOWLEDGMENTS

We would like to express our deep gratitude to all the people who supported us through the years to be good "macrobians" (people who follow macrobiotic principles) and to complete this book as our next step toward better macrobiotic cooking practices. Thank you!

Especially...

Our parents, Rodrique and Louise Lechasseur, the late Toshiko Suzuki and the late Shin Takashima. Without their love we would not be existing on this planet.

Our teachers, Michio Kushi and the fondly remembered Aveline Kushi, for their eternal dedication to Macrobiotic education.

Madonna for her continued passion for good food, health and in believing in our vision. Angela Becker for her care and kindness over the years.

Tobey Maguire for his support, and for his kind and honest feedback on our cooking.

Our photographer, Yoshi Ueda, for his patience and artistic vision.

Our graphic designers, Christine Goodreau and Mike Ellison, for their friendship and support since the beginning of our Macrobiotic learning and teaching process.

Our assistant, Doug Clayton, for continuing to help correct and edit our English and believe in our goals.

Our long time good friend, Judy Lee, always our English teacher.

Our organic garden keeper, Stephen Dorsey, for taking care of our "golden girls" and cats.

Our new student, Kimiko Miyazawa, for her infectious energy.

We appreciate our ceramicist friends...
Vladimira Zbori, for her dynamic and kind earthy energies. Michiko Nakamura, for her passion for ceramics. Yoriko Ikuzawa, for her playful arts.

And of course our four-legged family...
Three beautiful "golden girls," Kin, Dore and Kula, for their endless curiosity and patience no matter how long we take cooking and creating our recipes. As well as our two alley cats, Key-chain and Mai, for their honesty and proof that we can be who we really are no matter what circumstances we go through.

Thank you, thank you, and thank you
to you all and to this universe and this lifetime.
We are happy to have you all in our lives.

FOREWORD

Macrobiotics. When most people hear the word, they think of food. A diet. A strict set of rules relating to what you can and cannot eat. As a founder of the natural foods movement in the United States and after more than fifty years of dedication to a macrobiotic lifestyle, I can tell you that what you eat is only one element of achieving a lifestyle that is truly 'macrobiotic'. A discussion of how to create a healthy lifestyle may begin with choices of foods to eat, but then must also involve explorations of daily behavior, activities, and priorities. Macrobiotics, at its most fundamental level, is about balance. Eating all the 'prescribed' foods, but doing so at a cost to your own happiness and peace, would be counteractive to the benefits from the diet itself. *Love, Eric & Sanae* is written with an understanding of this principle, and gives you a selection of recipes and suggestions that are intended to encourage a manageable and energy-producing lifestyle.

Many people begin their macrobiotic journey due to a problem with their health. Cancer, allergies, injuries, and many other maladies can all encourage someone to examine themselves and begin making healing choices. In these times of illness and trial, we are willing to sacrifice our habits and our luxuries in order to heal and recover. A more difficult challenge faces us when the time comes for the transition from time of crisis to time of peace. When the initial problem is gone, how do we continue our macrobiotic practices in the long term? How can macrobiotics become a way of life, instead of a medical technique? This is a question often left unanswered in books on macrobiotics, which either focus on encouraging people to try macrobiotics for immediate health benefits, or provide vast amounts of knowledge on the subject for those who have already dedicated their lives to the practice.

In this cookbook by husband and wife team Eric Lechasseur and Sanae Suzuki, the authors open a window for us into their everyday lives. Eric and Sanae live in Santa Monica (near Los Angeles), and live lifestyles similar to many people living in America today - they have several jobs, many activities, and often have obligations that can make them very busy. Some days they are stressed and in trauma, while on others they find time to relax and enjoy the simple act of cooking their dinner. But no matter what the circumstances on any particular day, they rely on macrobiotics to maintain their health and give them energy to excel at whatever they do.

The recipes and comments in this book reflect the daily truth of their lives. Many of the recipes are very simple - efficient meals that can be prepared quickly for days when time is limited. Some can be prepared and kept in a box or container for when there is no time at all. There are also recipes for the days when the pressures of life are not heavily brought to bear, and time can be spent enjoying the act of cooking and savoring the delicious

FOREWORD

flavors and textures of the food itself. (I highly recommend the Tempeh Crab Cakes for an evening of relaxed culinary delight). In short, *Love, Eric & Sanae* is a cookbook for living. While some cookbooks you may use once a month or less, this is a book that will take up residence on your counter and refuse to leave it.

I met Sanae in the summer of 1994. She was volunteering with a group of Japanese students who were attending the Kushi Summer Conference that year. Some of the students were staying at my home in Brookline, and we met when she came by to talk with them. I warmed to Sanae right away. She had a wonderful balance of excitement about macrobiotics and respect for me and the other teachers. Her questions were always thoughtful and intelligent, and she seemed to have a never ending supply. In a remarkably short period of time, I developed a mentor relationship with her that continues to this day. At one point, my wife Aveline and I even invited Sanae to become my personal assistant. (She had just taken a position with Erewhon Natural Foods in Los Angeles, however, and was unable to accept. It was our loss).

I met Eric several years later at a macrobiotic fund-raising dinner for the Smithsonian Institute, where he and Sanae were volunteering as chefs for the event. At the time, Eric was still beginning his macrobiotic journey, having discovered it initially to help Sanae through a bout of cancer a few years before. Eric was already a very accomplished chef, particularly in French and Asian cooking styles, and was exploring how to incorporate his experience with the macrobiotic principles he was now aware of. Sanae was a health practitioner, on her way to earning certificates in massage therapy, shiatsu, herbology, and so on. I met Eric at this very exciting point in their lives when the two of them were learning to make macrobiotics a comfortable daily foundation to the rest of their studies.

Over the last decade since I first met them, I have watched their spirits grow in leaps and bounds, both individually and together. (They were married in June of 2004). Their dedication to fostering healing lifestyles for themselves and those around them has truly added to our world in innumerable ways. This book is only the most recent stop in a journey that began years ago, and that will continue to heal and grow those of us lucky enough to travel with them for a time.

Welcome to Eric and Sanae's world of daily macrobiotic living. I hope you become happier and more peaceful through your experience with them, as I have.

Michio Kushi
The world leader of Macrobiotic education
for health and peace
Brookline, Massachusetts

A NOTE FROM ERIC & SANAE

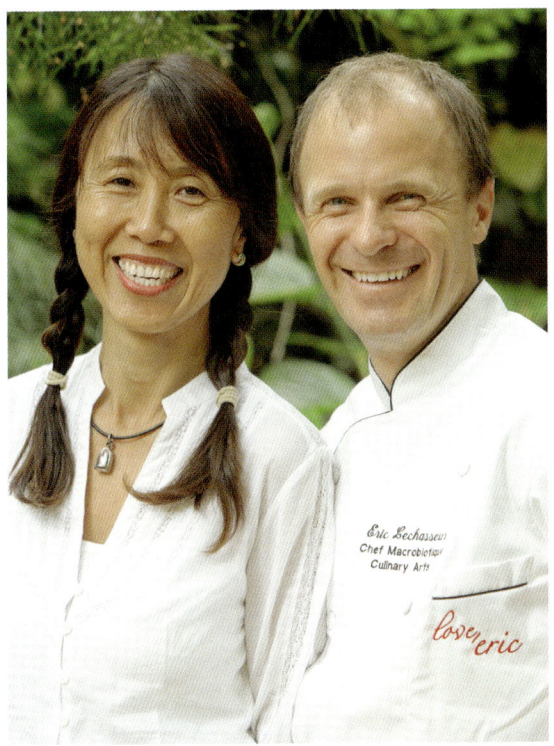

Many people begin the practice of macrobiotics with great enthusiasm, learning about the subject through books, study centers, and personal counselors. As hard as they work initially, a greater challenge awaits them when they try to maintain the practice of macrobiotics in their everyday lives, year after year.

Gradually the new excitement is gone, and ways must be found to make macrobiotic foods and philosophies feasible and practical. The noble end is suddenly overwhelmed with concerns about the means. 'It's harder than I thought.' 'It's so inconvenient.' 'It's too strict.' 'It takes too much time.' 'What are Yin and Yang, anyway?' In our world of super-fast and uber-convenient trends, investing the time and energy to truly follow macrobiotics seems frustrating and counterproductive.

When we began our macrobiotic journey, our purpose was to become more "healthy." We had several significant medical problems between the two of us, and we wanted them to go away. In this, we were similar to many people as they first look into macrobiotics, seeing it as a "magic diet" that can have "supernatural" healing effects. In the years since, however, we have come to realize that macrobiotics is not just how we eat, but how we live. It is not just about strict rules of what to eat and what not to eat, but more importantly it is also a practice of choosing healthful foods,

A NOTE FROM ERIC & SANAE

activities, and ways of behaving that support our individual conditions, needs, lifestyles, and environment. It is about balance and positiveness, as much as it is about avoiding processed foods.

We live in Santa Monica, California, adjacent to Hollywood and Beverly Hills. Los Angeles is overwhelmed with stress and harsh stimulants from traffic jams, smog, chemical products, pressure to achieve artificial beauty and health, and a culture that insists on rushing everywhere. As macrobians (people who follow macrobiotic principles), it is difficult to maintain balance and live in this sort of environment. But we also value the beauty to be found here as well. Santa Monica Canyon, Topanga, and the Pacific Ocean are a few examples of the natural beauty that fill us daily. We are also blessed to be close to so many outdoor activities. We can ski in the morning and watch the sunset over the ocean at night, or surf at dawn and then hike in the mountains all day. Even the city itself, on a day when the air is clear, can be an inspiring and fulfilling sight.

We are also blessed to have beautiful organic produce and grains available at all times for us to create our delicious macrobiotic foods.

We appreciate the balance between the things we have and those that we don't, which is exactly the teaching of "Yin and Yang" that macrobiotics is all about. Appreciation and acceptance, however, are not enough. Anything in life that is worth doing or worth learning about takes an investment of energy. If you refuse to ever take the time to learn, you would never have learned how to sing or play the piano, never ridden a bike or skied, or never learned to cook anything more complicated than a TV dinner. It is the importance to your life or to your heart that pushes you to dedicate yourself to these pursuits. You have to drive to get around, so you practice until you learn how. Your love and passion for playing the piano keep you going, even when you sound terrible and grow frustrated. It is the same with any activity you need to do, or that you are passionate about doing.

Cooking is the same, a pursuit that requires love and dedication to fully realize. Unfortunately, in the last thirty years since the invention of frozen convenience foods and the microwave oven, cooking has rapidly become a disregarded activity. These days many people do not cook at all, choosing instead to "prepare" a prefabricated meal, or for even more convenience, opt for fast food. We no longer care about what we put in our mouths, as long as it's edible, fills our tummies, and satisfies our taste buds with increasingly intense and artificial flavors.

We feel that as a culture we need to re-recognize several things. First, what our food is for. The food we eat literally forms our bodies. It generates the blood, muscle, skin, and bones that comprise us and produces the energy required to power our movements and thoughts. Second, cooking takes time, and creating quality food that will be beneficial to our bodies in the most effective way will take more time than throwing something together. Like anything worth doing, the invested time is more than balanced by the benefits we receive.

These two ideas, though simple to state, are difficult to incorporate into the daily lifestyles which most of us have. This makes the pursuit of macrobiotics, or any other healthy eating practice, a lifelong learning experience. We have created this cookbook with a desire to help those of you on this journey take a few more steps down the road to healthy living.

This cookbook is not an all-encompassing tome of macrobiotic recipes. Instead, it is a window into our lives as regular people who live a macrobiotic lifestyle, day in and day out. Some days we don't have any time at all, so we make the simplest of recipes. On other days, our time is more free, and we can savor the experience of cooking and eating throughout the entire day. Every day is different, and the food we create reflects that. These recipes show a sampling of the dishes that are the foundation stones to our everyday meals. Your lifestyle may be different than ours. Please feel free to experiment and be flexible based on how you live and how you feel. Following these recipes strictly is not the goal if it goes against what you feel strongly in your heart. These are only suggestions to help you further your own quest for health and wholeness.

No one likes getting sick. No one likes pain and suffering. But like any difficulty, illness prompts us to take action to improve ourselves. Our lives have benefitted immeasurably from macrobiotics and other healthy practices, which we would never have pursued if not for all the traumas we have experienced. In this way, we feel fortunate to have had our health problems, and to have the daily challenges that confront us. They have ushered us to not only health, but the freedom to live a life we enjoy and to feel true happiness.

We hope that this book helps you on your journey, and that you may find a life as happy as the one we have.

Love, Eric & Sanae
Santa Monica, CA

Have you ever really thought about why spring is called "spring"? We often think of winter as still, quiet and dormant. Then, one day we notice things beginning to change. Life bursts forth and everything starts growing, lifting and "springing" upwards!

Spring is our favorite season (and the season of our birthdays), so we have a tendency to bounce and leap and be over-energized. We must remember to slow down and not miss the beauty of the opening cocoons and the first blossoms of the season.

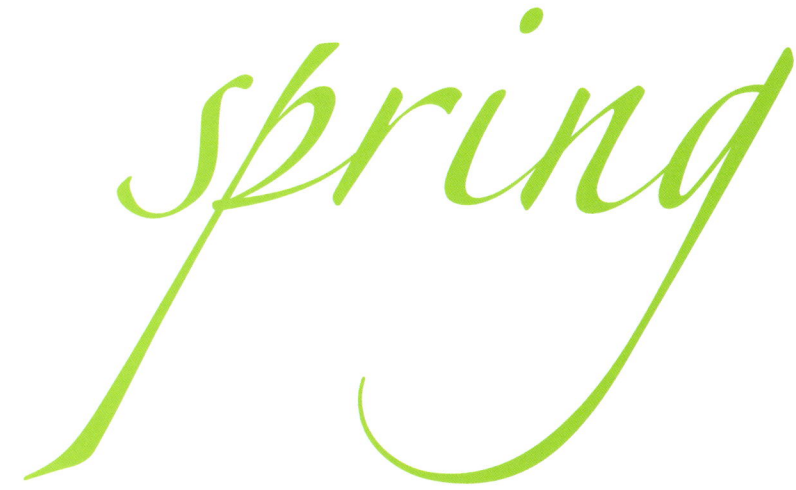

spring

Carrot and Garbanzo Soup with Lotus Root and Dill

Kombu Dashi

Leek and Cauliflower Filo Wrap with Mint Sauce

Country Whole Barley with Fava Beans

Pressed Wakame and Napa Cabbage Rolls

Tempeh Crab Cakes with Caper Sauce

Sautéed Pea Sprouts

Strawberry Cupcakes

Apricot Linzer

Green Tea with Chamomile

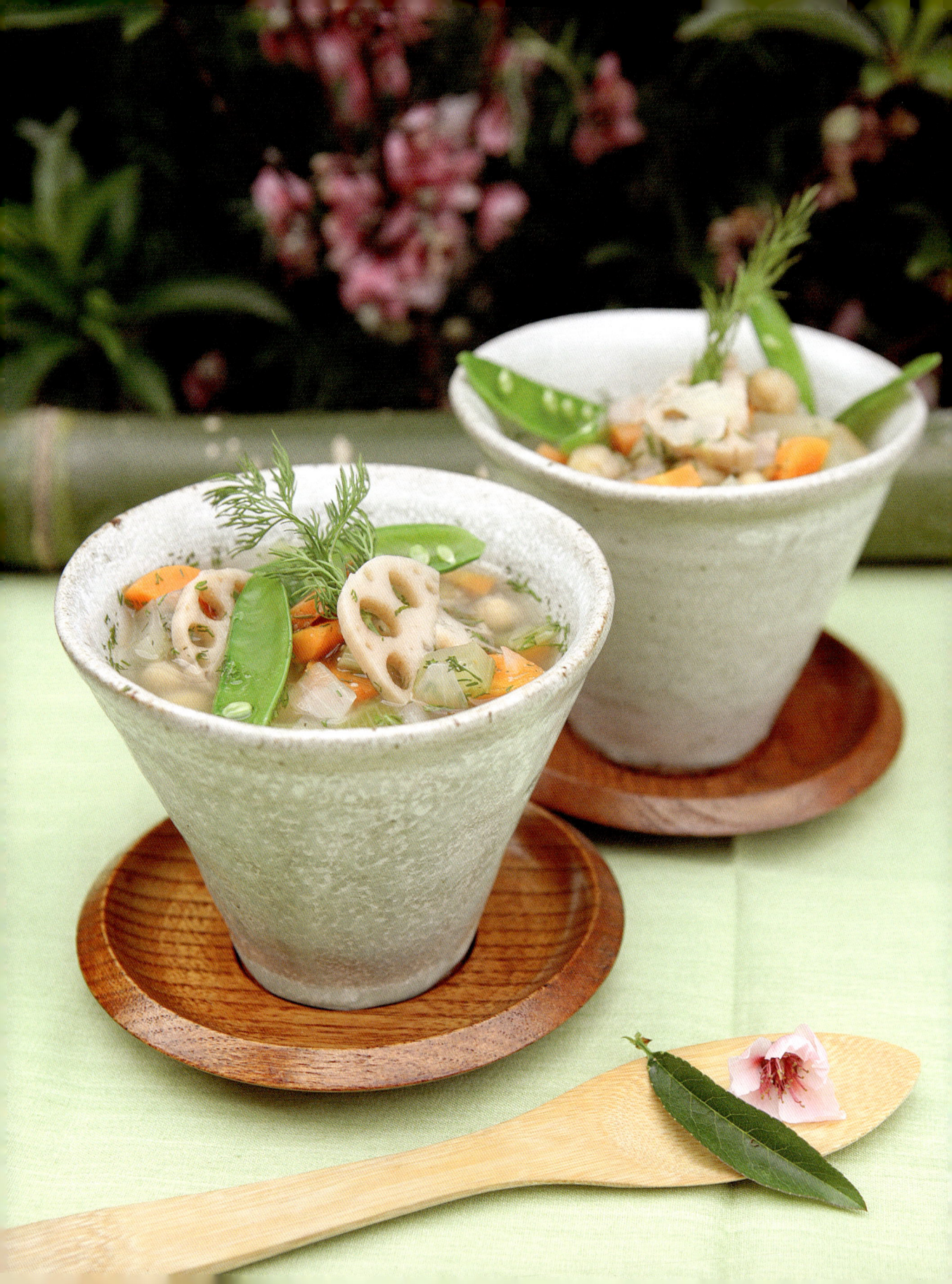

SPRING — LOVE, ERIC & SANAE

Carrot and Garbanzo Soup
with Lotus Root and Dill

Spring is the season when the first batch of sweet baby carrots arrive! The addition of garbanzos makes this a hearty dish.

MAKES 4 SERVINGS

For the garbanzo beans:
½ cup garbanzo beans, sorted and rinsed
purified water for soaking
4 cups purified water for cooking
1-inch strip of kombu

For the soup:
½ onion, diced
4 cups kombu dashi (see recipe below)
3 carrots, diced
2 stalks celery, diced
¼ cup lotus root, sliced
1 tablespoon white miso
¼ cup dill, chopped
¼ cup sugar snap peas, blanched

To make the garbanzo beans:
1. Soak the beans in ample water for 4 to 6 hours. Drain.
2. In a large pot with a lid, combine the beans, water and kombu and bring to a boil.
3. Cover and simmer for 45 minutes, or until beans are fully cooked and still retain their shape.

To make the soup:
1. In a large saucepan over medium heat, sauté the onions with ½ cup kombu dashi until onions become translucent. Add the carrots, celery and lotus root, and cook for a few more minutes.
2. Add the garbanzo beans and the balance of the kombu dashi. Simmer for 20 minutes.
3. Remove from heat, stir in the miso and chopped dill.
4. Pour into individual bowls and serve garnished with sugar snap peas.

Kombu Dashi

This is a basic recipe for the mineral-rich broth commonly used in Japanese soups. Several recipes from this book require this easy-to-make flavor-enhancing stock.

For the dashi:
purified water
kombu (use one 1-inch square piece per cup of water)

To make the dashi:
1. Wipe the kombu clean with a dry cloth.
2. No-cook method: Soak the kombu in the water for 2 to 3 hours.
   Stovetop method: In a saucepan, bring the water and kombu to a boil, reduce heat, and simmer for 20 to 30 minutes.
3. Strain to remove the kombu. Dashi will keep for 2 or 3 days in the refrigerator.

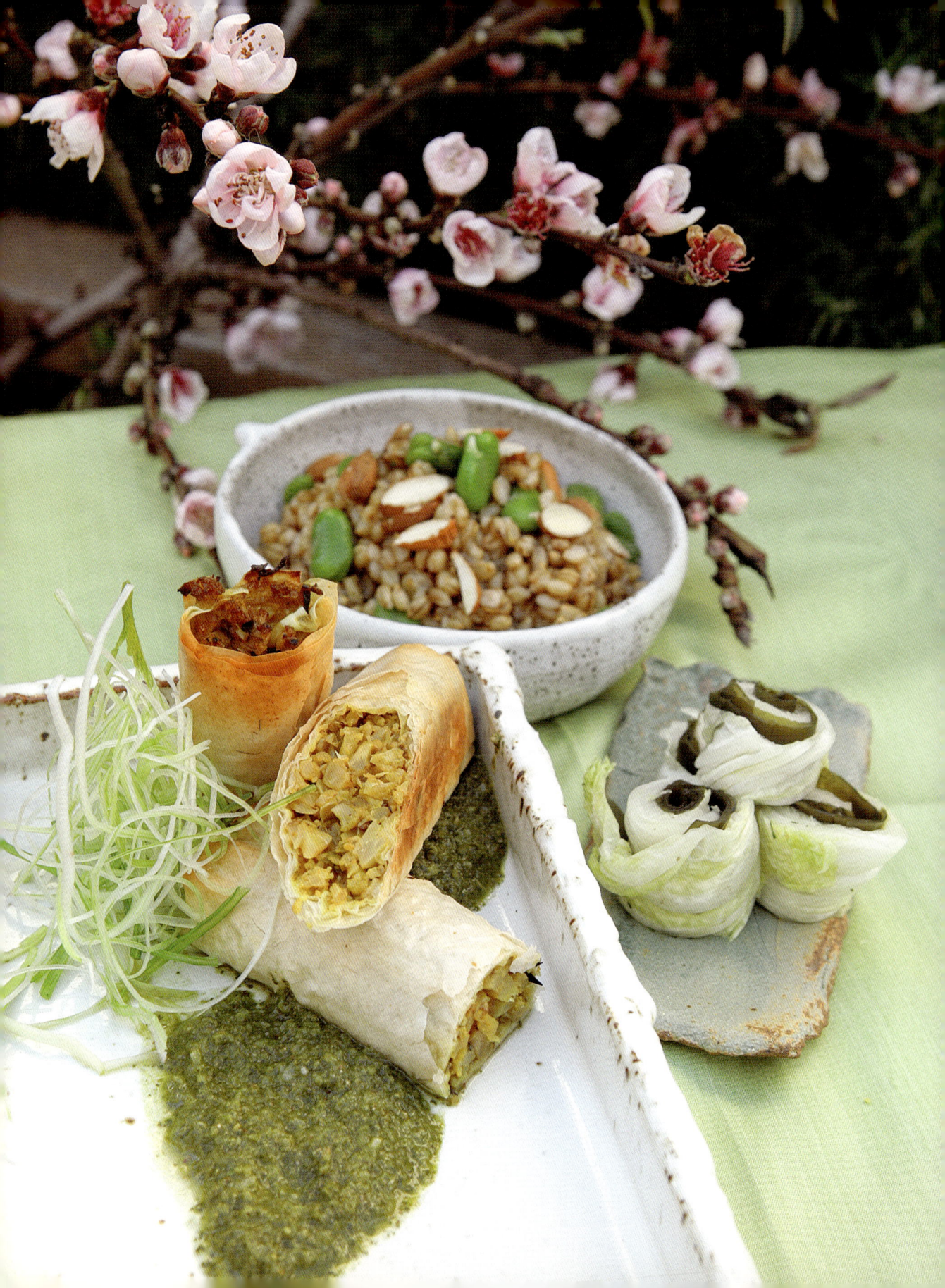

leek and cauliflower filo wrap
with Mint Sauce

One of our favorite cuisines is East Indian. Even without the potatoes, this cauliflower wrap will satisfy your cravings for Indian flavors. The uplifting sweetness of leeks is a perfect energizer for the spring season.

MAKES 4 SERVINGS

For the sauce:
¼ cup onions, chopped
¼ cup mint, chopped
¼ cup cilantro, chopped
1-inch piece ginger, chopped
juice of 1 lemon
2 tablespoons water
1 teaspoon coriander powder
2 tablespoons safflower oil

For the wraps:
2 tablespoons olive oil
1 leek (white part), thinly sliced
2-inch piece of ginger
1 small cauliflower, chopped
1 teaspoon caraway seeds
2 pinches turmeric powder
3 sheets whole grain filo dough
¼ cup olive oil, for brushing filo dough sheet

To make the sauce:
1. In a blender, combine all ingredients and purée until smooth.
2. Sauce will keep for up to 2 days in the refrigerator.

To make the wraps:
1. Preheat the oven to 400° F.
2. In a skillet, warm the oil over medium heat. Sauté the leeks and ginger until translucent. Add the cauliflower and cook for a few more minutes.
3. Stir in the caraway seeds and the turmeric powder. Cook for a few more minutes.
4. Cover and continue cooking for an additional 8 to 10 minutes. Remove from heat and allow to cool.
5. Using a potato masher, lightly mash the mixture.
6. On a flat surface, lay out 1 sheet of filo dough and brush lightly with oil. Lay a second sheet over the first and brush again. Repeat with the final sheet of filo dough.
7. Cut the filo dough into four equal pieces. Separate the cauliflower into four equal portions.
8. Spoon a portion of the cauliflower along the edge of each piece of filo dough and roll up.
9. Place the wraps on a baking pan lined with parchment paper, and bake for 15 to 20 minutes.
10. Serve wraps with Mint Sauce on the side.

SPRING — LOVE, ERIC & SANAE

country whole barley
with Fava Beans

A tasty spring harmony is created when the chewy heartiness of barley is combined with the tenderness of freshly cooked fava beans.

MAKES 4 SERVINGS

For the grains and beans:
½ cup whole barley
½ cup short grain brown rice
2 cups purified water for the grains
1 pinch sea salt for the grains
2 pinches sea salt for the beans
2 cups fresh fava beans, removed from pods
¼ cup roasted almonds, coarsely chopped

To make the grains and beans:
1. Combine the barley and rice in a mesh strainer. Place strainer in a bowl under cold running water and rinse until the water is clear, usually three times or more. Drain. Transfer the grains to a 5-quart pan with a lid, add the purified water and soak for 4 to 6 hours.
2. Add the pinch of sea salt, bring to a boil, cover and simmer for 50 minutes. Remove from heat and set aside.
3. Meanwhile, in a 2-quart saucepan, blanch the fava beans in boiling salted water. Plunge beans in ice water and drain. Peel the thick "skins" off of each bean and set aside.
4. Transfer cooked grains to a large bowl. Thoroughly combine the fava beans with the grains. Stir in the almonds and serve.

pressed wakame and napa cabbage rolls

This simple dish of wakame sea vegetable and napa cabbage is very versatile and is a wonderful complement to any spring meal.

MAKES 4 TO 6 SERVINGS

For the rolls:
4 to 5 strips of wakame
8 napa cabbage leaves
2 teaspoons sea salt

To make the rolls:
1. Soak the wakame in water for 10 minutes and drain. Cut out the larger center veins if needed.
2. In a large bowl, combine the cabbage, sea salt and wakame and stir by hand for about one minute.
3. Transfer to a pickle press* and press for 2 hours.
4. Rinse the pickles to reduce excess saltiness, if necessary. Roll cabbage leaves with wakame and slice into bite-sized pieces.
5. Rolls will keep for several days in the refrigerator.

*see equipment list on page 90

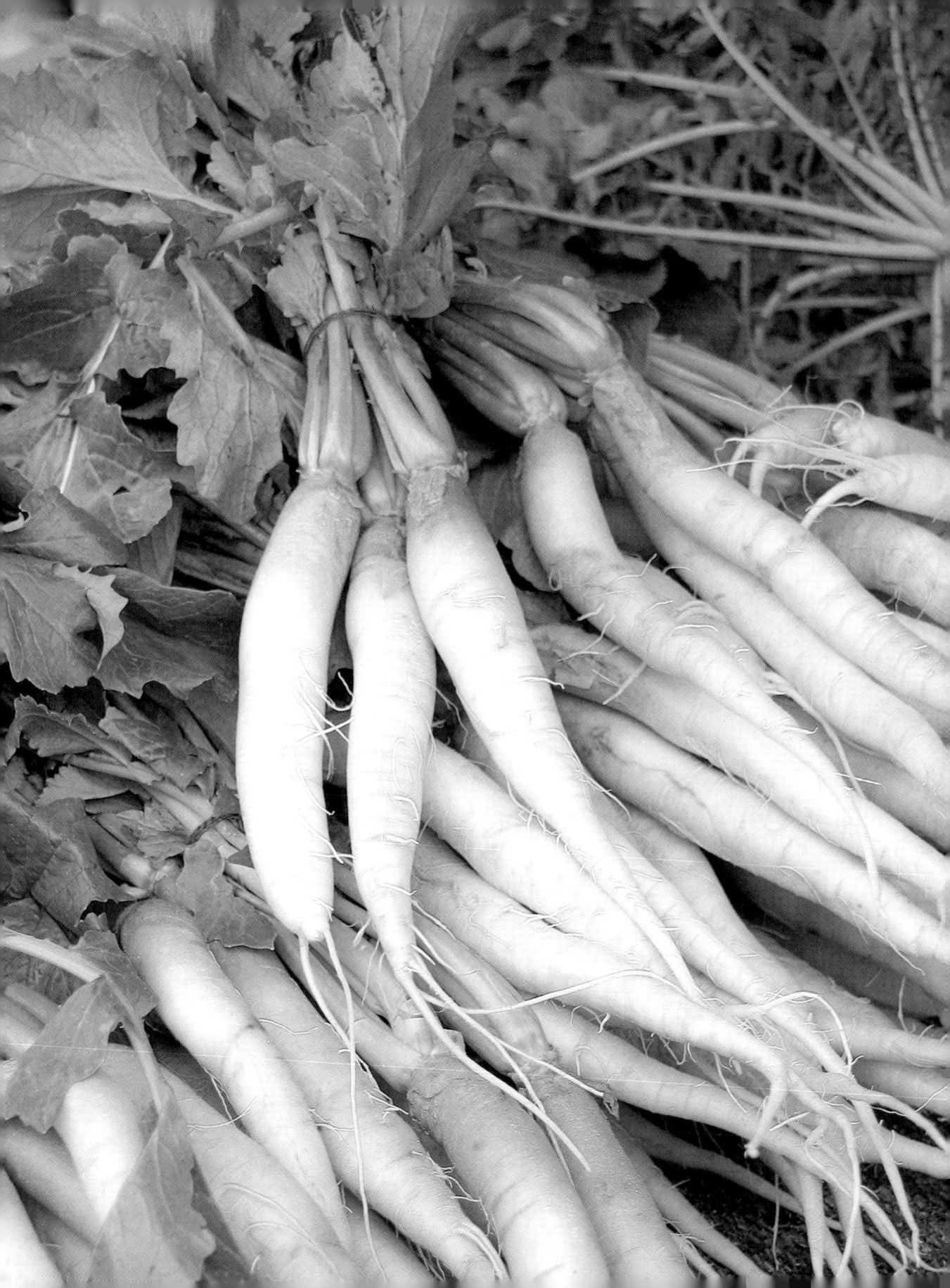

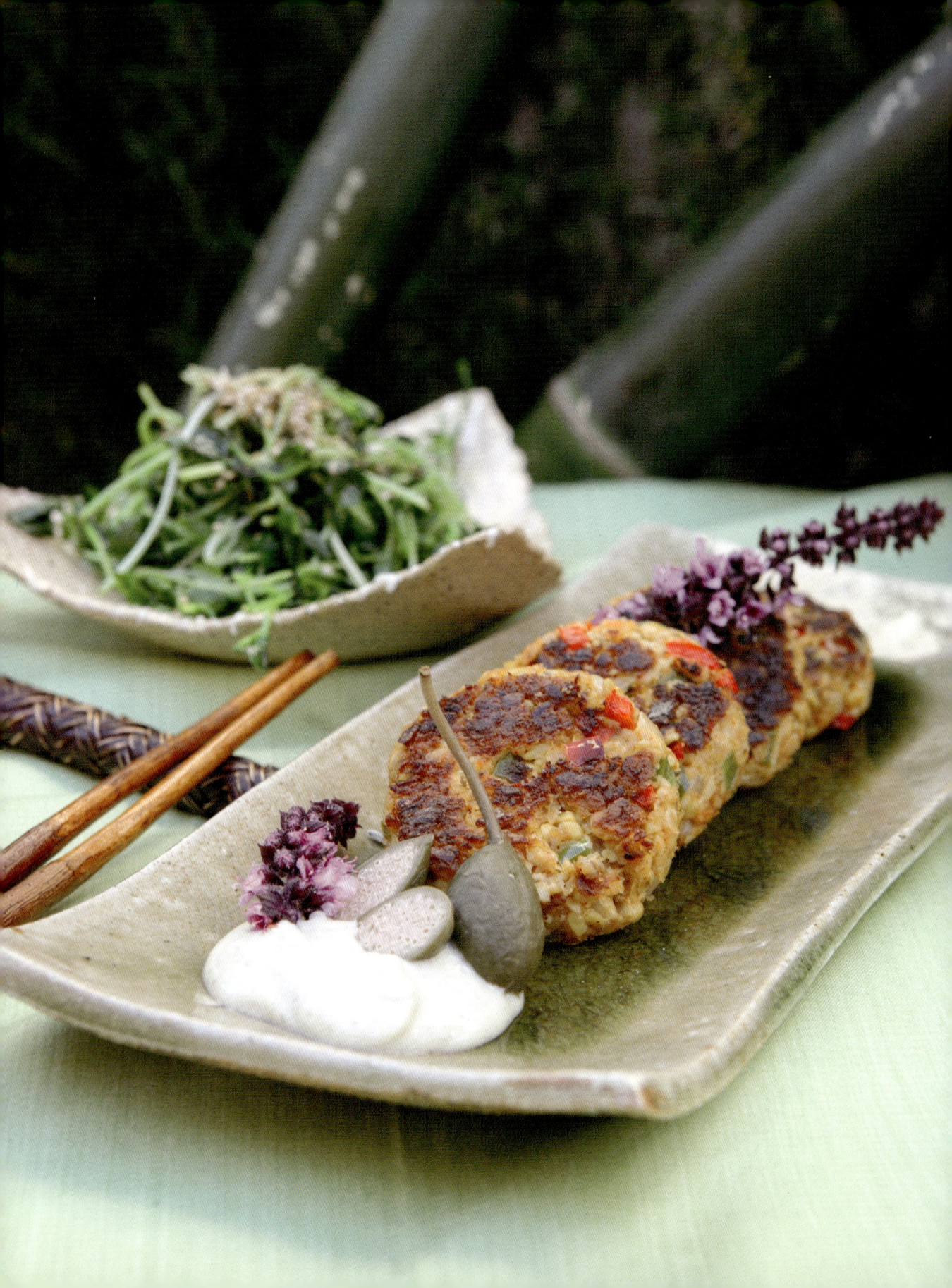

tempeh crab cakes
with Caper Sauce

This is quite a dish! It's one of our most popular recipes. Even friends who have never tasted tempeh before ask for seconds. Try it for yourself and enjoy!

MAKES 4 SERVINGS

For the sauce:
2 tablespoons capers
3 ounces tofu
¼ cup olive oil
1 tablespoon rice syrup
2 pinches sea salt
1 tablespoon parsley, chopped

For the tempeh cakes:
8 ounces tempeh
1 tablespoon olive oil
¼ onion, chopped
¼ cup red pepper, chopped
¼ cup green pepper, chopped
1 clove garlic, chopped
½ cup sourdough bread crumbs
½ teaspoon paprika
1 teaspoon oregano
4 tablespoons Vegenaise

To make the sauce:
1. In a blender, combine the capers, tofu, olive oil and rice syrup and mix well. (You can use a hand mixer, if you prefer.)
2. Transfer to a bowl, stir in the sea salt and parsley, and refrigerate until ready to use.
3. Sauce will keep for up to 2 days in the refrigerator.

To make the tempeh cakes:
1. Slice the tempeh into 8 pieces and steam for 10 minutes.
2. In a large skillet over medium heat, warm the oil. Sauté the onions, peppers, and garlic for a few minutes. Transfer the mixture to a large bowl.
3. Add remaining ingredients and stir well. Allow to cool and form mixture into 8 patties.
4. Sauté patties in a lightly-oiled skillet over medium-high heat for a few minutes on each side, until golden brown.
5. Serve immediately with Caper Sauce on the side.

sautéed pea sprouts

Nothing says "spring" quite like sprouts! These sprouts sauté quickly so it's almost like you're enjoying a fresh, raw salad.

MAKES 4 SERVINGS

For the sprouts:
1 teaspoon sesame oil
½ pound fresh pea sprouts
2 pinches sea salt

To make the sprouts:
1. In a wok over high heat, warm the oil.
2. Add the sprouts and sea salt and sauté for just 1 minute or less. Serve hot.

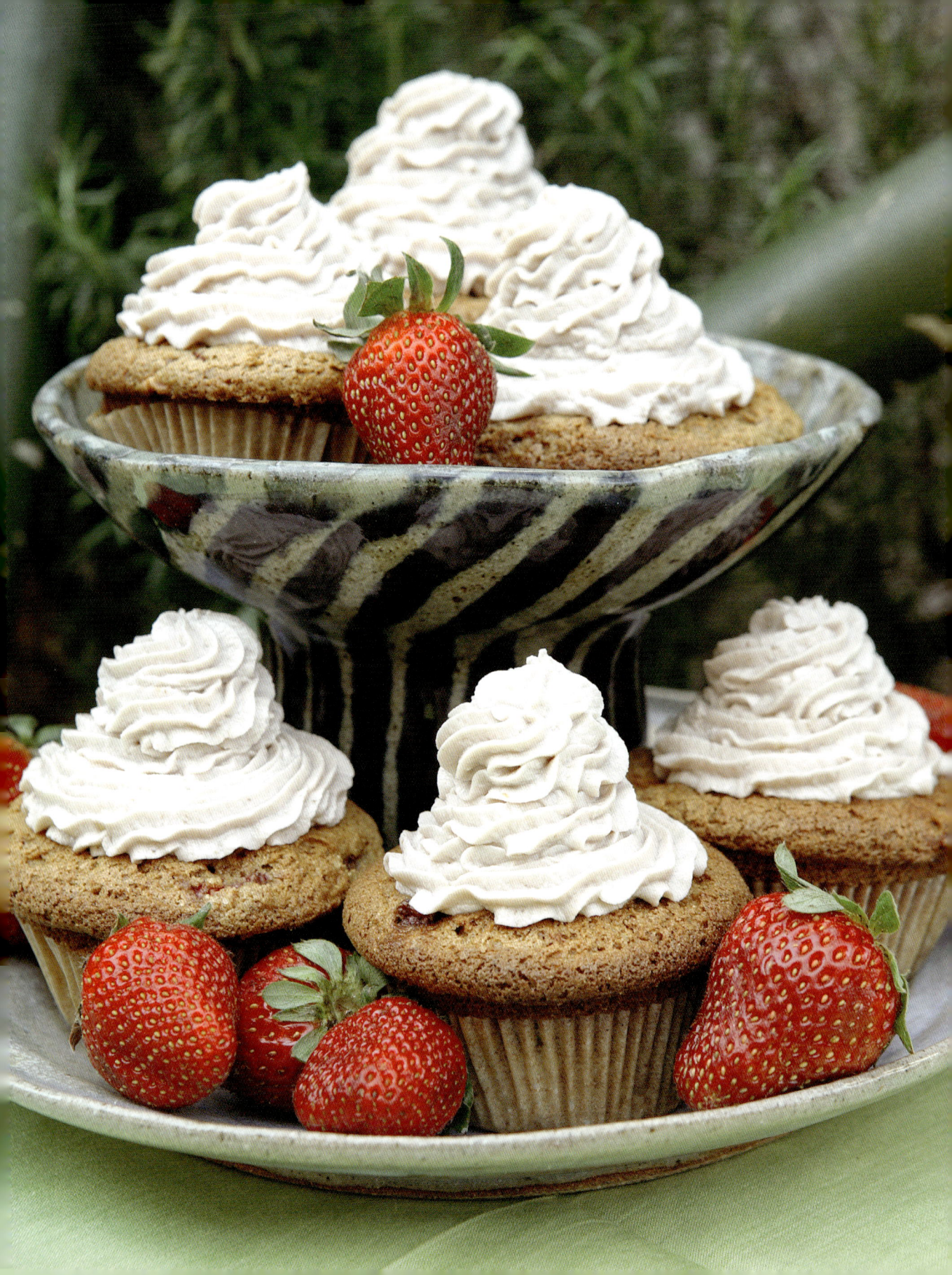

Strawberry Cupcakes

Who doesn't love cupcakes? Especially these beautiful creations with freshly-picked spring strawberries.

MAKES 12 CUPCAKES

For the cupcakes:
1 ⅓ cups white spelt flour
1 ¼ cups oat flour
1 pinch sea salt
2 teaspoons baking powder
2 teaspoons baking soda
¾ cup maple syrup
⅓ cup safflower oil
⅓ cup soy milk (unsweetened)
½ teaspoon vanilla extract
4 ounces silken firm tofu

For the frosting:
14 ounces extra firm tofu
1 teaspoon vanilla extract
¼ cup maple syrup
5 ounces fresh organic strawberries
2 tablespoons agar flakes
⅓ cup water
¼ cup safflower oil

To make the cupcakes:
1. Preheat the oven to 325° F.
2. In a large bowl, combine the flours, sea salt, baking powder and baking soda.
3. In a blender, combine the maple syrup, oil, soy milk, vanilla and tofu. Blend until smooth.
4. Pour the tofu mixture into the flour mixture and combine gently with a wire whisk.
5. Divide into 12 muffin cups and bake for 30 minutes.
5. Remove cupcakes from oven and allow to cool.

To make the frosting:
1. In a food processor, combine the tofu and vanilla and purée until very creamy and smooth.
2. Add the maple syrup and purée again. Transfer mixture to a bowl and set aside.
3. Purée the strawberries separately. Add the tofu mixture and purée again.
4. In a saucepan over medium-low heat, simmer the agar with the water until dissolved. Add to the strawberry tofu mixture and purée until well combined.
5. In a small saucepan, warm the oil to 80° F and slowly pour into the food processor while it is mixing. This step ensures a creamy-textured frosting.
6. Allow frosting to cool and spread over the top of each cooled cupcake.

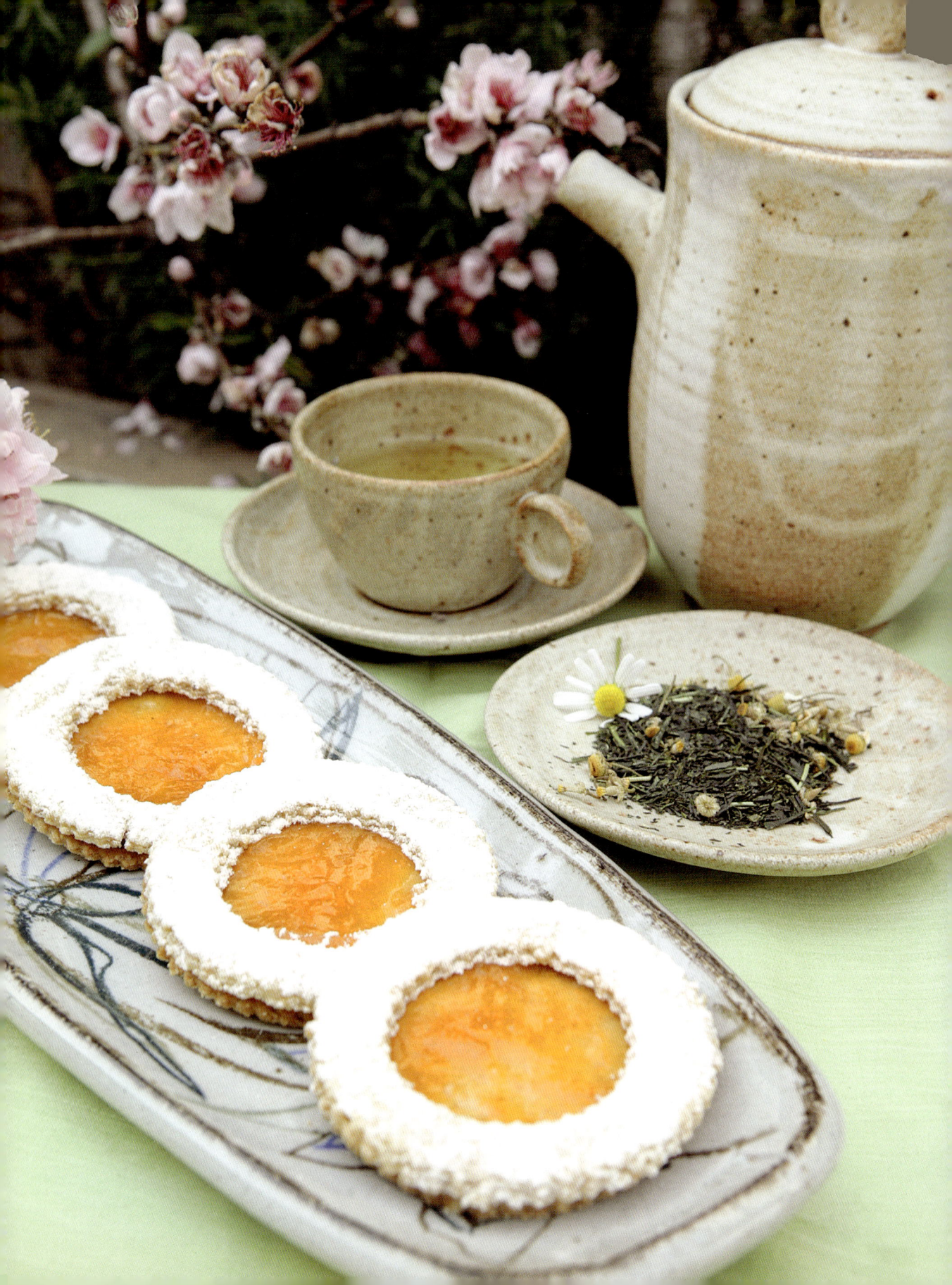

SPRING — LOVE, ERIC & SANAE

apricot linzer

These cookies look and taste so luscious — who would think they are Macrobiotic? Apricot jam is not a common choice, but try it for variety's sake, and you'll know why we picked apricots!

MAKES 12 COOKIES

For the cookies:
1 cup slivered almonds
1 cup rolled oats
1 cup whole grain pastry flour
½ teaspoon baking powder
1 pinch sea salt
¼ cup safflower oil
¼ cup maple syrup
1 teaspoon vanilla extract
4 ounces unsweetened apricot jam
powdered coconut (as needed)

To make the cookies:
1. Preheat the oven to 350° F.
2. In a food processor, process the almonds to a powdered consistency, being careful not to over mix into an almond butter. Add the oats and process again until lightly coarse.
3. Add the pastry flour, baking powder and sea salt. Process for a few seconds and transfer to a bowl.
4. In a small bowl, whisk the oil, maple syrup and vanilla.
5. Add the oil mixture to the flour mixture and knead well.
6. Divide the dough into two halves. Using a rolling pin, one-at-a-time roll each dough piece between 2 sheets of parchment paper to form a ¼-inch thick rectangle. Peel away top layer of parchment.
7. Using a 3- to 4-inch cookie cutter, cut the dough into 12 shapes and remove the excess dough. Use a smaller cookie cutter to cut a hole in the center of 6 of the cookie rounds — leaving the other 6 intact and set aside. Repeat the rolling and cutting process with the second half of the dough.
8. Slide the parchment paper containing the cookies onto a baking sheet and bake for 12 minutes.
9. Allow cookies to cool. Spread the jam on the full cookie rounds, and place the donut-shaped round on top, making a sandwich. Sprinkle with powdered coconut.

green tea
with Chamomile

We like to add fresh chamomile from our garden to mellow out the caffeine. It also makes for an attractive cup of tea.

MAKES 2 CUPS

For the tea:
2 heaping teaspoons Ryokucha (green tea) leaves
a few fresh chamomile flowers
2 cups purified water

To make the tea:
1. Bring water to a boil. Add tea leaves to a teapot.
2. Pour the boiled water over tea leaves and allow to steep for 2 to 3 minutes.
3. Strain, add fresh chamomile flowers, and serve hot.

Look at the sky *in summer — it's so close, it seems like you could reach out and touch it. The sun is bright and very near.*

You feel like you can do anything in summer, and as a result you tend to do too much. You are dominated by the fire energy of the season.

We don't want to burn up, so we take a nap in the midday summer heat and sip cool barley or corn tea to soothe our heart chakra.

summer brunch

Honeydew Melon Soup

Vegetable Pancakes with Tofu Sour Cream

Inca Quinoa and Mustard Greens Salad

Zucchini Muffins

Scrambled Tofu Florentine with Hollandaise Sauce

Dulse and Cucumber with Basil

Grilled Nectarines with Lemon and Maple Glaze

Hazelnut Baci

Cool Roasted Corn Tea

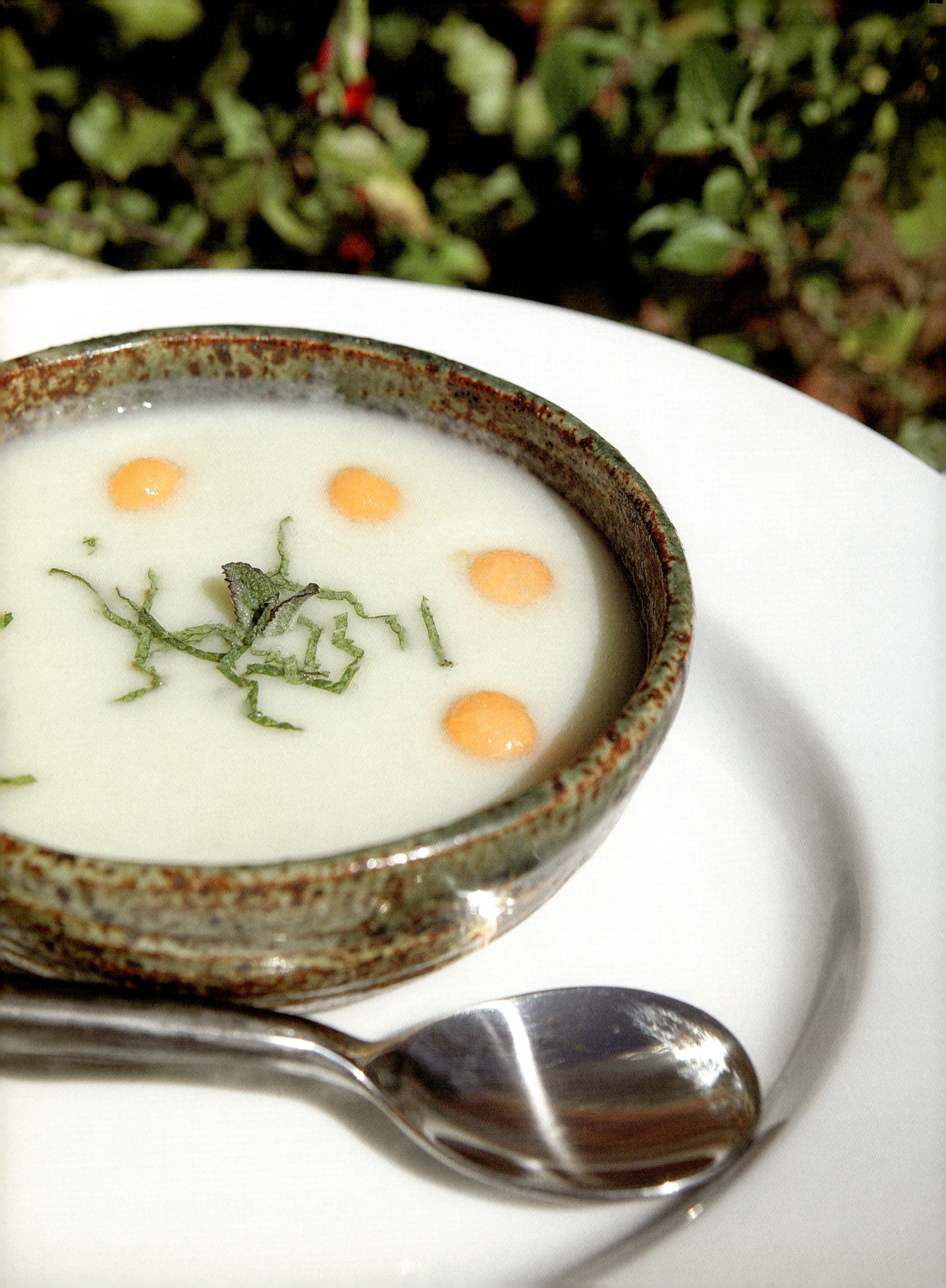

honeydew melon soup

Honeydew is our favorite summer melon, not only for its name, but for the smooth, sweet taste that melts in our mouth. This is a delightful choice for a cool summer soup.

MAKES 4 SERVINGS

For the soup:
1 honeydew melon
6 ounces soy yogurt (unsweetened)
1 pinch sea salt
freshly ground white pepper (if desired)
2 fresh mint sprigs
½ cantaloupe

To make the soup:
1. Using a knife, peel the skin from the honeydew melon. Slice the melon in half, remove the seeds, and chop coarsely into pieces.
2. In a blender, purée the honeydew melon, soy yogurt, sea salt, and pepper until smooth.
3. Transfer to a large container and refrigerate for a few hours.
4. Using a melon ball scoop, form balls from the cantaloupe flesh and set aside.
5. To serve, pour soup into individual bowls, and garnish with the melon balls and fresh mint.

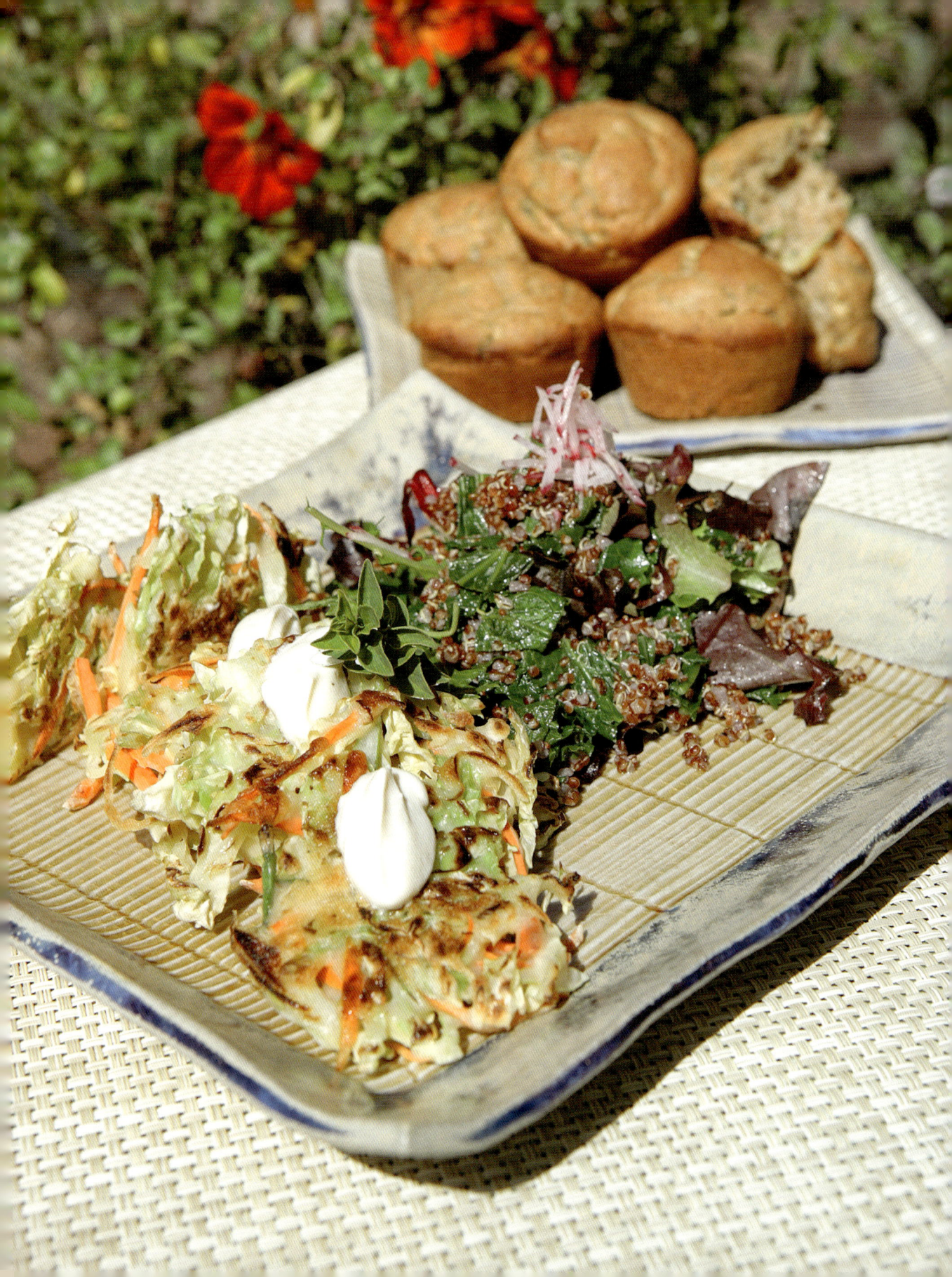

vegetable pancakes
with Tofu Sour Cream

These light, fluffy, savory pancakes, served with tofu sour cream, give sweet breakfast pancakes a run for their money.

MAKES 4 SERVINGS

For the tofu sour cream:
6 ounces silken tofu
juice of 1 lemon
2 pinches sea salt
2 tablespoons olive oil

For the pancakes:
1 cup cabbage, shredded
¼ cup onion, sliced
1 carrot, shredded
4 scallions, sliced
2 cups unbleached flour
½ teaspoon sea salt
1 teaspoon baking powder (optional)
1 teaspoon kudzu
¾ cup rice milk (unsweetened)
4 tablespoons green nori flakes
safflower oil, for frying

To make the tofu sour cream:
1. In a blender, combine all the ingredients and blend until creamy.
2. Transfer to a container and refrigerate until well chilled. Will keep for up to 2 or 3 days in the refrigerator.

To make the pancakes:
1. In a large sauté pan over medium heat, quickly "water sauté"* the cabbage, onion, carrot and scallions. Set aside and allow to cool.
2. In a large bowl, combine the flour, sea salt and baking powder.
3. In a small bowl, dissolve the kudzu in the rice milk. Add to the flour mixture. Using a wire whisk, stir lightly to form a batter.
4. Add the cooked vegetables and nori flakes to the batter and gently fold together.
5. In a large lightly-oiled skillet over medium-high heat, pour the batter in 2-ounce drops.
6. Cook for a few minutes on each side, until golden brown.
7. Serve immediately with a dollop of Tofu Sour Cream.

To water sauté:
In a stainless steel skillet, place enough water to just cover the bottom of the pan and bring to a boil. Add the vegetables to sauté.

inca quinoa and mustard greens salad

Fresh baby greens are beautiful to taste in the summer, and when combined with mustard greens and heirloom Inca quinoa grains, they're sure to be the hit of the party!

MAKES 4 SERVINGS

For the dressing:
juice of 2 lemons
1 teaspoon maple syrup
¼ cup olive oil
2 pinches sea salt
freshly crushed black pepper (optional)

For the salad:
1 cup red quinoa
2 cups water
1 pinch sea salt
1 bunch mustard greens, coarsely chopped
2 ounces mixed baby greens

To make the dressing:
1. In a small bowl, combine all the ingredients using a wire whisk.
2. Transfer to a container and refrigerate.

To make the salad:
1. In a medium saucepan, combine the quinoa, sea salt and water.
2. Bring to a boil and simmer for 20 minutes. Allow to cool and set aside.
3. In a medium sauté pan, water sauté the mustard greens for a few minutes, drain well, and allow to cool.
4. In a large serving bowl, combine the quinoa, baby greens, and mustard greens. Toss salad with the dressing and serve.

zucchini muffins

Our vegetable muffins are very lightly sweetened, so you can enjoy them as part of a meal, instead of for dessert.

MAKES 12 SERVINGS

For the muffins:
1 cup spelt flour
1 tablespoon baking powder
1 pinch sea salt
½ cup zucchini, shredded
¾ cup rice milk (unsweetened)
¼ cup safflower oil
¼ cup maple syrup

To make the muffins:
1. Preheat the oven to 350° F.
2. In a large bowl, combine the flour, baking powder, sea salt and zucchini.
3. In a separate bowl, using a wire whisk, combine the rice milk, oil and maple syrup.
4. Add the liquids to the flour and whisk lightly.
5. Pour 4 ounces of batter in each cup of an oiled muffin pan.
6. Bake for 30 minutes or until a toothpick inserted into the center of a muffin comes out clean. Allow to cool slightly before serving.

SUMMER BRUNCH — LOVE, ERIC & SANAE

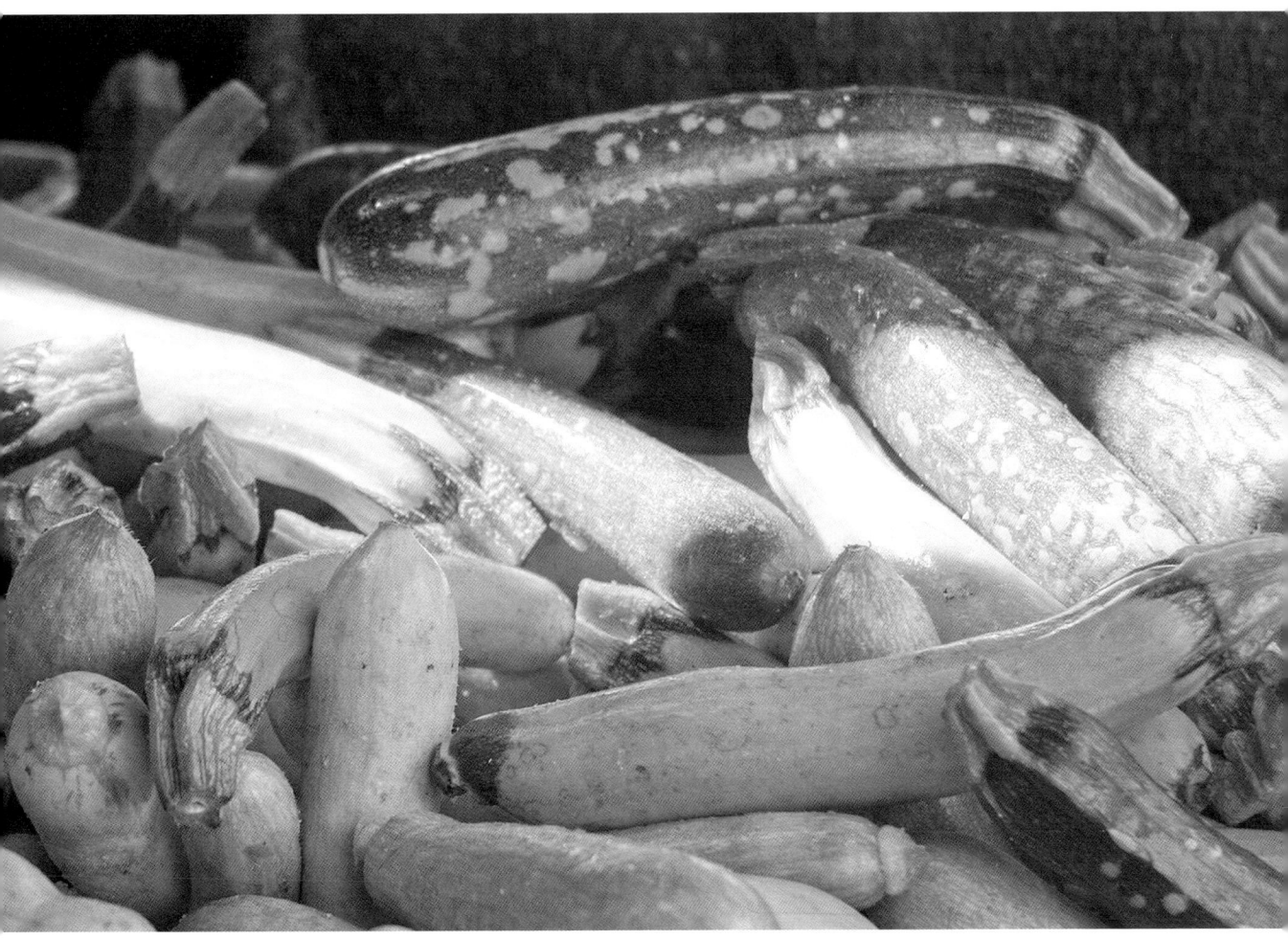

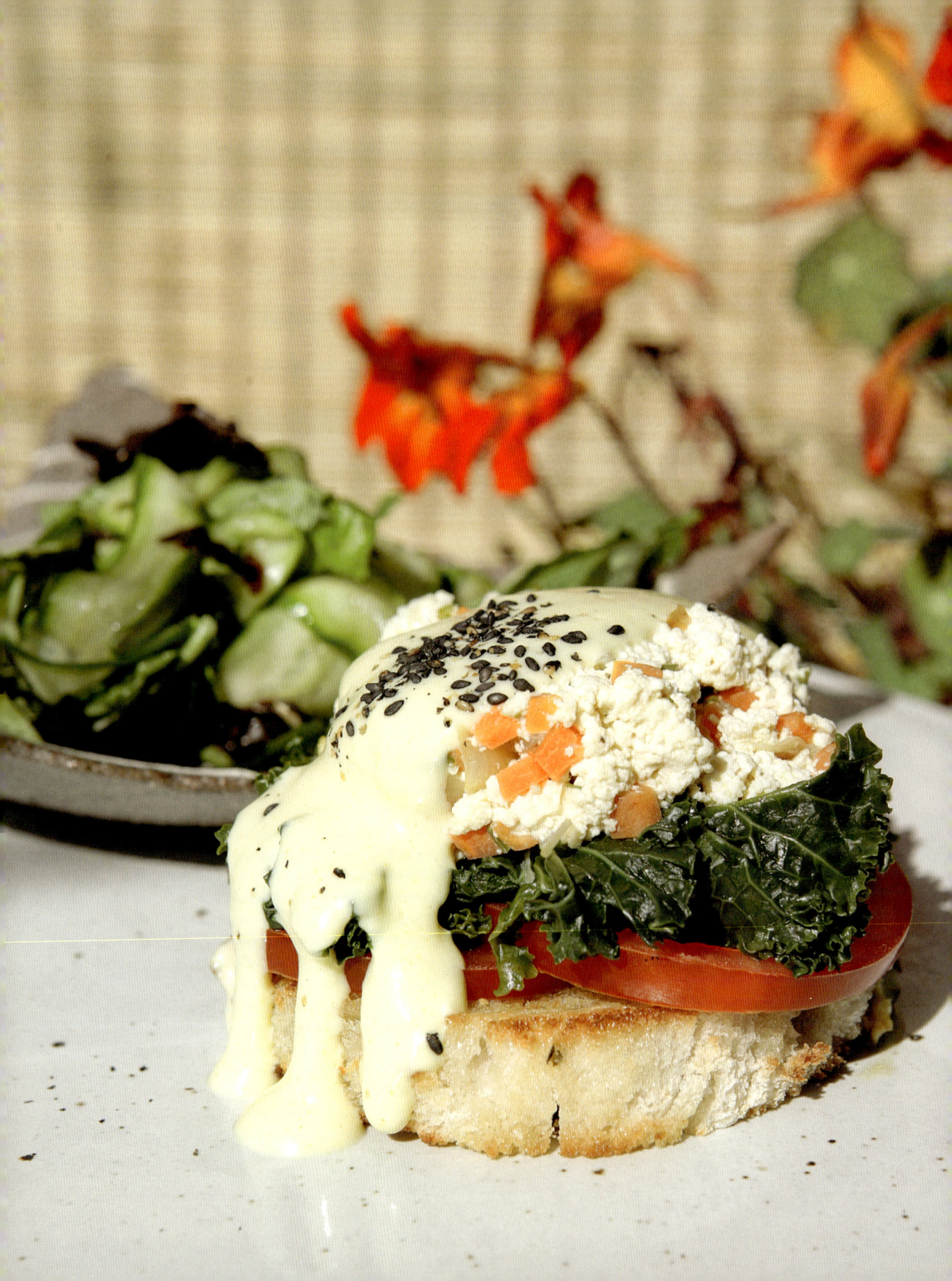

Scrambled tofu florentine
with Hollandaise Sauce

Tofu has come a long way from traditional Asian cuisine to a dish like this, which will pleasantly surprise people who think they don't like tofu.

MAKES 4 SERVINGS

For the sauce:
6 ounces silken firm tofu
1 teaspoon Dijon mustard
¼ cup Vegenaise
½ cup olive oil
2 pinches turmeric
juice of 1 lemon
2 pinches sea salt
¼ cup rice milk (unsweetened)

For the tofu:
12 ounces firm tofu
1 tablespoon olive oil
½ cup onion, chopped
½ cup carrot, diced
1 pinch turmeric
sea salt and crushed pepper as needed
4 pieces sourdough bread, lightly toasted
4 to 6 slices tomato (optional)
1 bunch kale, chopped and blanched

Optional garnish:
black sesame seeds, roasted

To make the sauce:
1. In a blender, combine all the ingredients and blend until very creamy.
2. Set aside.

To make the tofu:
1. Crumble the tofu by hand and set aside to drain in a mesh strainer.
2. In a large skillet, warm the oil. Add the onions and carrots, and sauté until onions become translucent.
3. Add the tofu, turmeric, salt and pepper, and cook over a medium-high flame for about 5 minutes, stirring continuously.
4. Remove from heat and set aside.

To assemble:
1. Place one piece of bread in the center of each plate. Stack a slice of tomato and a portion of the chopped kale on each piece of bread.
2. Add the tofu scramble and top with hollandaise sauce.
3. Garnish with sesame seeds and serve.

dulse and cucumber
with Basil

Most people ask us, "What's dulse?" With its beautiful burgundy color and sea-salty taste, dulse is a sea vegetable harvested in Northern California. Enjoy this perfect pressed salad on a hot summer day.

MAKES 4 SERVINGS

For the salad:
1 to 3 cucumbers (Japanese or Persian), thinly sliced
½ ounce dulse
4 to 6 fresh basil leaves

To make the salad:
1. Scissor cut or tear the dulse into bite-sized pieces.
2. In a medium bowl, combine all the ingredients and transfer to a pickle press* for 20 to 30 minutes.
3. Remove pickles from press and rinse if they taste too salty. Squeeze out excess liquid by hand and serve. Pickles will keep for up to 3 days in the refrigerator.

see equipment list on page 90

SUMMER BRUNCH — LOVE, ERIC & SANAE

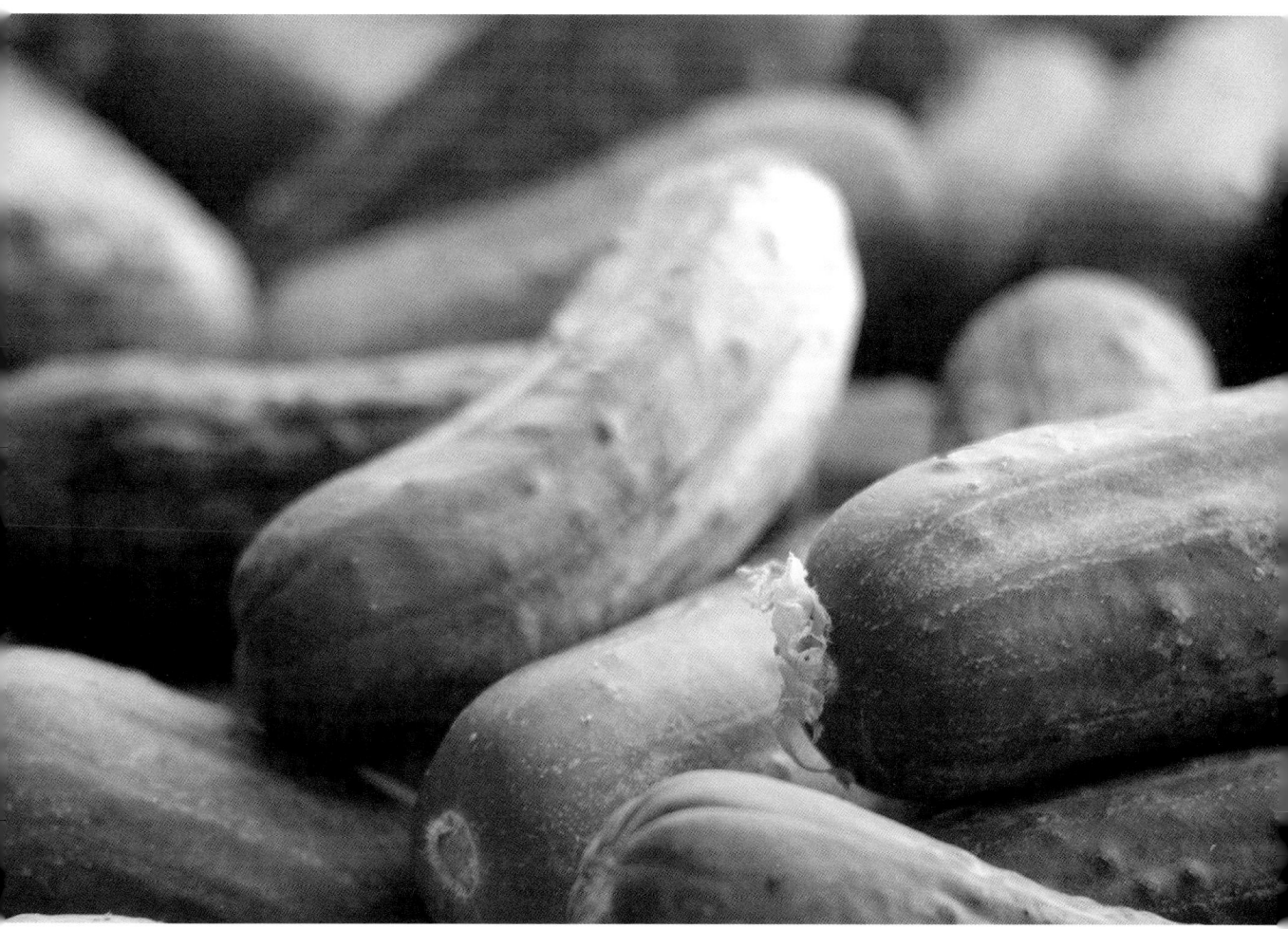

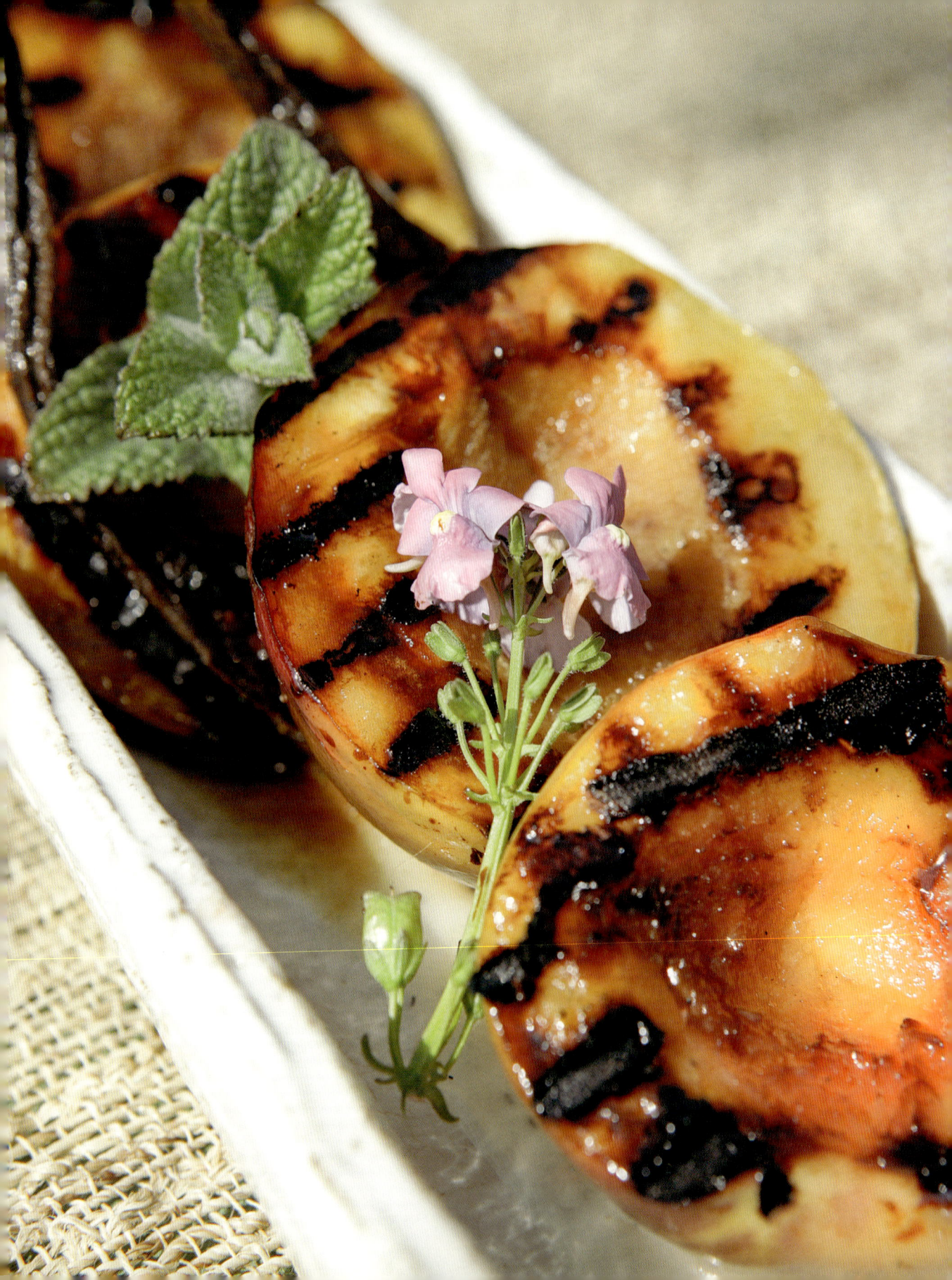

grilled nectarines
with Lemon and Maple Glaze

Everybody in America loves a barbecue in the summer. How about barbecued fruits as desserts? It's so easy and tasty.

MAKES 4 SERVINGS

For the nectarines and glaze:
4 fresh nectarines, sliced in half
juice of 1 lemon
2 tablespoons olive oil
1 pinch sea salt
¼ cup maple sugar

To make the nectarines and glaze:
1. In a small bowl, combine the lemon juice, oil and sea salt. Brush all sides of the nectarines with the lemon juice and oil mixture.
2. Sprinkle the maple sugar on the cut side of each nectarine, and allow to sit for 15 minutes.
3. Grill or pan fry the nectarines. Serve warm or at room temperature.

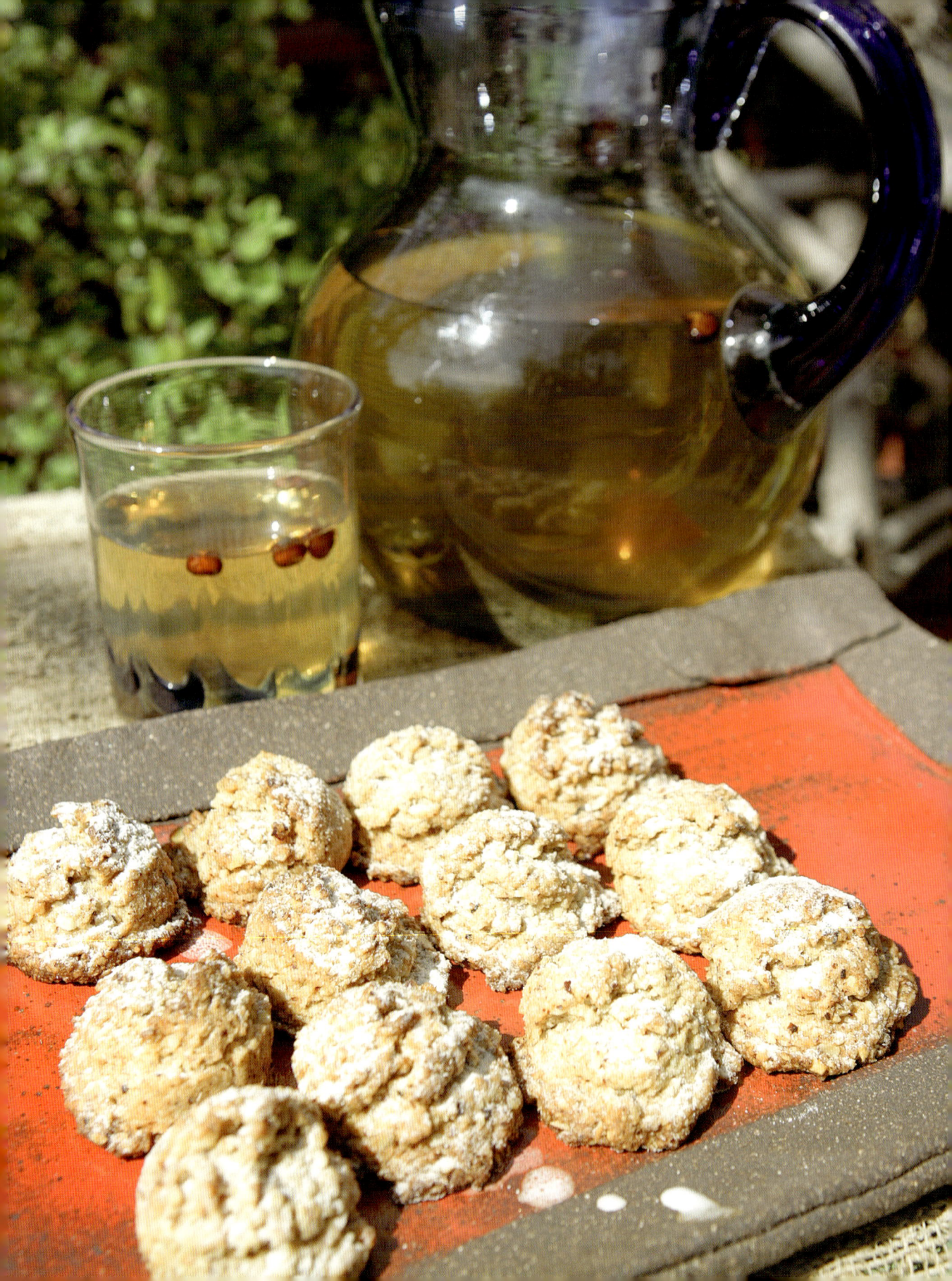

SUMMER BRUNCH — LOVE, ERIC & SANAE

hazelnut baci

These nutty, grainy confections are scrumptiously addictive!

MAKES 20 TO 25 COOKIES

For the cookies:
1 cup hazelnuts
1 cup rolled oats
1 cup whole wheat pastry flour
¼ teaspoon baking powder
2 pinches sea salt
⅓ cup safflower oil
½ cup maple syrup
1 teaspoon vanilla extract
powdered rice syrup

To make the cookies:
1. Preheat the oven to 375° F.
2. In a food processor, grind the hazelnuts until they turn into a fine meal. Transfer to a large bowl.
3. In a small bowl, whisk together the oil, maple syrup and vanilla extract.
4. Add the oats, flour, baking powder and salt to the powdered hazelnuts and stir well to combine.
5. Add wet ingredients to dry and stir to combine.
6. Using a 2-ounce ice cream scoop, drop dough onto a baking sheet lined with parchment paper. Bake for 12 to 15 minutes.
7. Allow cookies to cool and dust with powdered rice syrup.

cool roasted corn tea

Sweet roasted corn makes a lovely tea with a very mild and refreshing taste.

MAKES 2 SERVINGS

For the tea:
4 teaspoons dry roasted corn kernels*
   (available at Asian and Latin markets)
2 cups purified water

To make the tea:
1. In a small saucepan over a medium-high flame, simmer dry-roasted corn in the water until liquid turns a light brown (about 5 minutes).
2. Allow to cool and serve. Strain before serving, if desired.

*If you wish to roast your own corn:
spread fresh corn kernels on a baking sheet and bake at 225° F for approximately 2 hours or until kernels turn brown.

This is the season that most of us don't know, since it isn't one of the traditional four, but this is a very precious and important time. Late summer gives us time to say "good-bye" to the exciting and active summer, and "hello" to the creative and calming seasons ahead.

Even in sunny Santa Monica we notice summer passing and can feel that it is a very sensitive time. As the vibrancy fades in nature, we notice the change and sense that we are a part of, and that we are, nature.

late summer

Sweet Corn Chowder with Basil Oil

Kamut Spaghetti with Pine Nuts and Sun Dried Tomatoes

Simmered Turnips

Arame Poppyseed Rolls

Stuffed Shiitake Mushrooms with Millet and Kudzu Beet Sauce

Melon and Thai Basil Pickles with Lemongrass

Pistachio Chocolate Mousse

Mini Blueberry Scones

Kukicha with Rose Hips and Petals

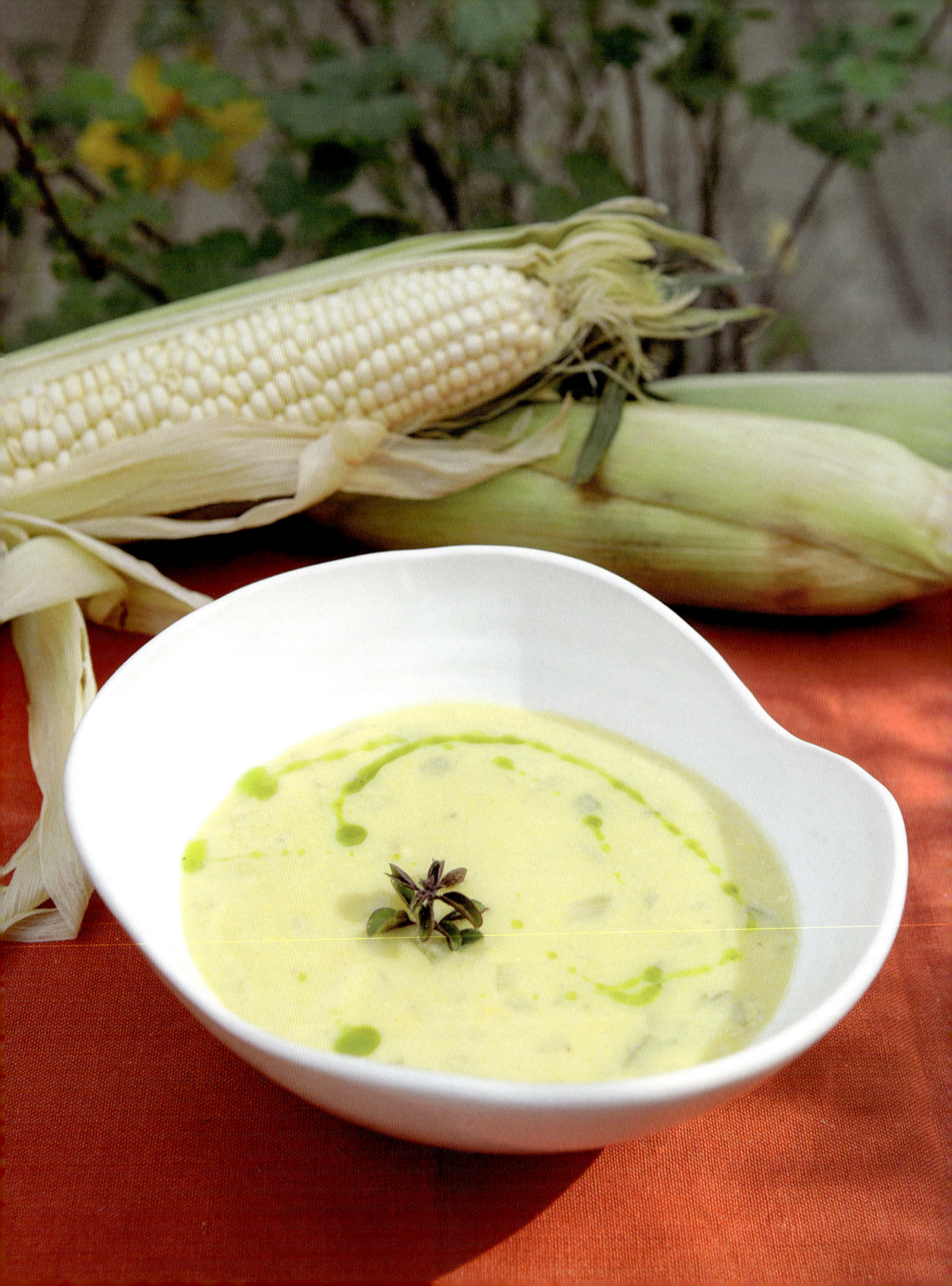

Sweet Corn Chowder
with Basil Oil

Late summer is peak season for fresh corn, so why not indulge in nature's bounty!

MAKES 4 SERVINGS

For the basil oil:
1 bunch fresh basil
¼ cup extra virgin olive oil

For the soup:
½ onion, diced
2 celery sticks, diced
1 pinch sea salt
3 cups kombu dashi (recipe on page 15)
kernels from 3 or 4 ears of fresh corn
½ potato, diced
1 teaspoon white miso

To make the basil oil:
1. Quickly blanch the basil in boiling water. Plunge in ice water and lightly towel dry.
2. In a blender, combine the basil and the oil and purée until smooth. Transfer to a container with a narrow pour spout and set aside.

To make the soup:
1. In a soup pot, combine the onion, celery, sea salt, and ¼ cup of the kombu dashi. Sauté on a high flame for a few minutes.
2. Add the corn, potatoes, and remaining kombu dashi.
3. Bring to a boil and simmer for 15 minutes.
4. Dissolve the white miso in the soup and simmer for 5 more minutes.
5. In a blender, purée half of the soup and pour back into the pot. Stir to combine.
6. Pour soup into individual serving bowls and garnish with drizzled basil oil.

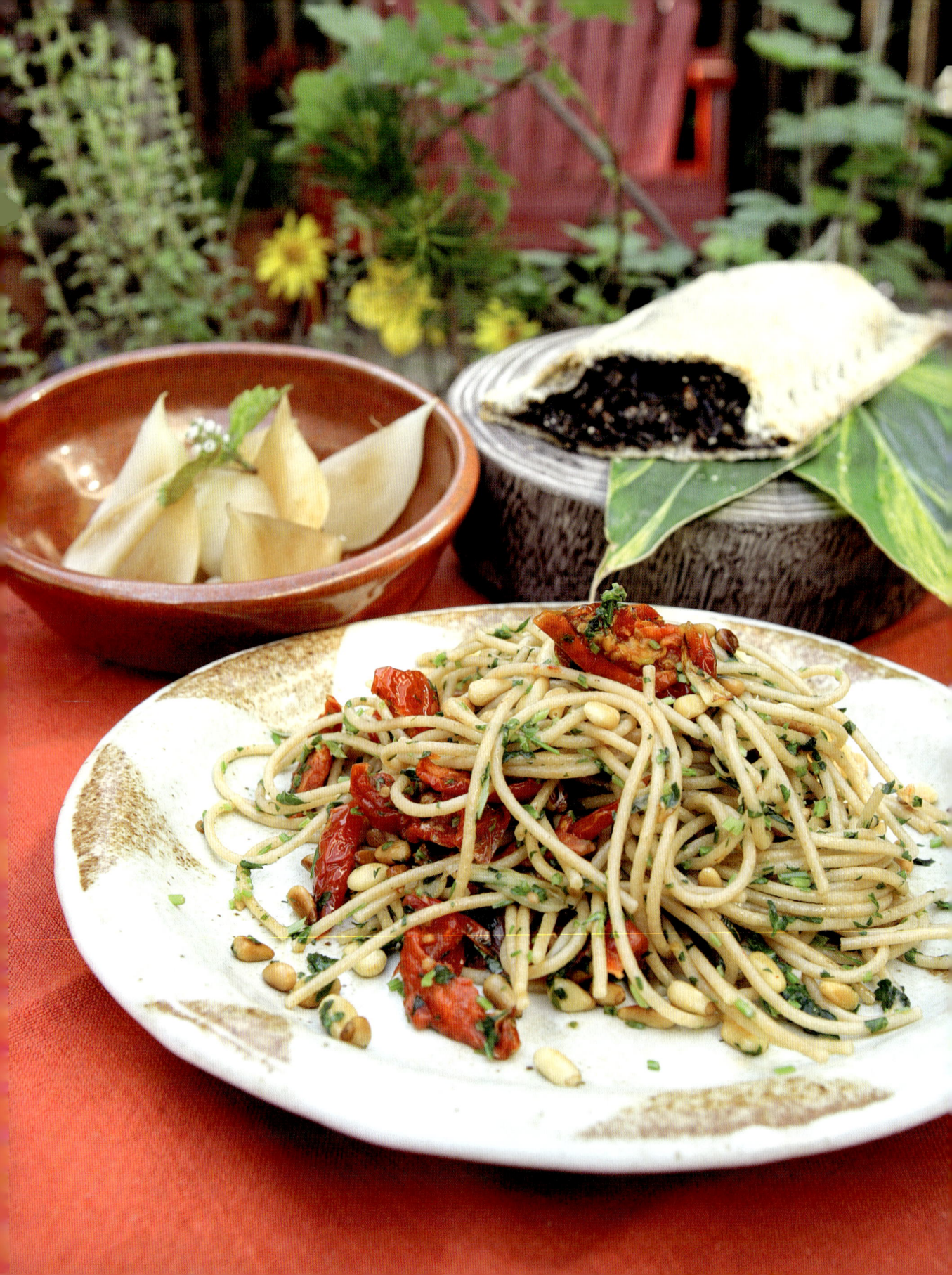

Kamut spaghetti
with Pine Nuts and Sun Dried Tomatoes

Pasta is our favorite dish on a tight schedule. It's quick and easy. This simple yet beautiful pasta is perfect for busy macrobians.

MAKES 4 SERVINGS

For the spaghetti:
1 12- to 16-ounce package organic Kamut spaghetti
1 pinch sea salt
1 tablespoon olive oil
½ cup sun dried tomatoes
½ cup roasted pine nuts
½ cup parsley, chopped

To make the spaghetti:
1. Bring a large pot of water to a boil.
2. Add the sea salt and cook the pasta to taste. Drain well.
3. In a large pan, warm the oil. Sauté the sun dried tomatoes, pine nuts and parsley for 1 minute.
4. Stir in the pasta, combine well, and season to taste.

Simmered turnips

Many of us forget the beauty and complexity of flavor in a simply prepared turnip. This recipe perfectly embodies the principles of macrobiotics.

MAKES 4 SERVINGS

For the turnips:
4 to 5 turnips
1 strip of kombu, about 3 x 7 inches
1 cup purified water
½ teaspoon soy sauce

To make the turnips:
1. Slice each turnip into 4 to 6 wedges, depending on the size of the turnips.
2. In a large sauté pan, combine the turnips, kombu and water. Simmer for 15 minutes.
3. Add the soy sauce and simmer a few minutes more, or until turnips are tender.

arame poppyseed rolls

If you are wary about eating sea vegetables, this recipe is for you. The mild flavor of arame is a wonderful introduction to the mineral-rich world of vegetables from the sea. You can enjoy this dish like a savory pie.

MAKES 4 TO 6 SERVINGS

For the arame:

½ cup arame
2 cups purified water, plus ¼ cup purified water
½ brown onion, thinly sliced
1 carrot, shredded
2 teaspoons soy sauce

For the dough:

⅔ cup whole wheat pastry flour
⅔ cup unbleached flour
4 tablespoons poppyseeds
1 pinch sea salt
2 ounces safflower oil
½ cup cold water

To make the arame:

1. Soak the arame in 2 cups of the water for 5 minutes. Drain and set aside.
2. In a medium saucepan, sauté the onions and carrots with ¼ cup of the water for a few minutes.
3. Add the arame. Cover and simmer for 20 minutes.
4. Add the soy sauce and cook for 5 more minutes. Allow to cool and set aside.

To make the dough:

1. Preheat the oven to 375° F.
2. In a large bowl, combine the flours, poppyseeds, and sea salt.
3. Add the oil to the dry mixture and stir gently with a fork.
4. Add the cold water and continue mixing gently to form a dough.

To make the rolls:

1. Divide the dough in half and roll each piece out to about 6 x 18 inches.
2. Brush the edges of the dough with water. Place half of the arame along the center of each piece of dough. Fold each piece of dough over to cover the arame, and seal the edges with a fork.
3. Place stuffed dough on a baking pan lined with parchment paper, and bake for 20 minutes.
4. Cut rolls to desired size and serve warm.

LATE SUMMER — LOVE, ERIC & SANAE

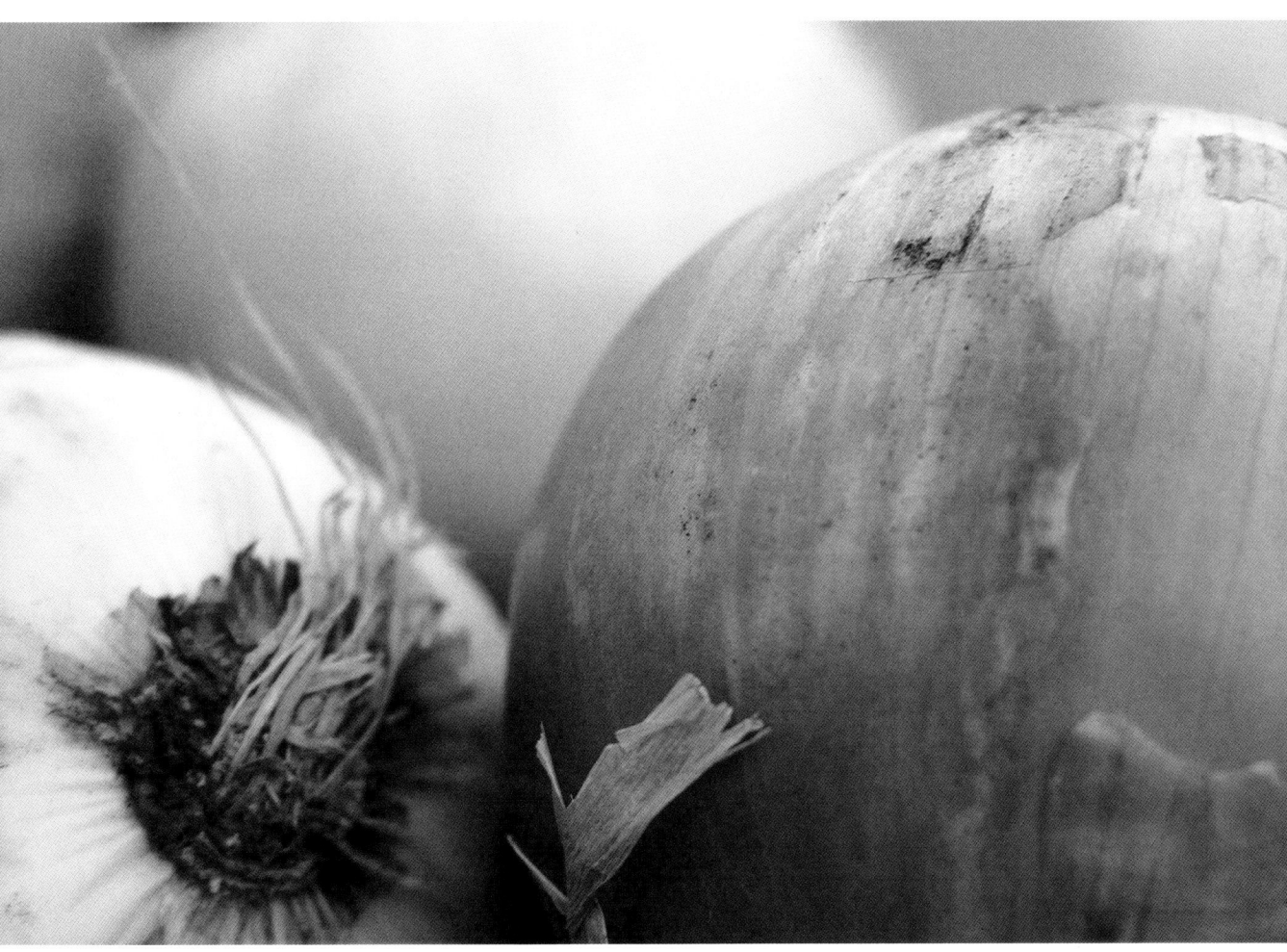

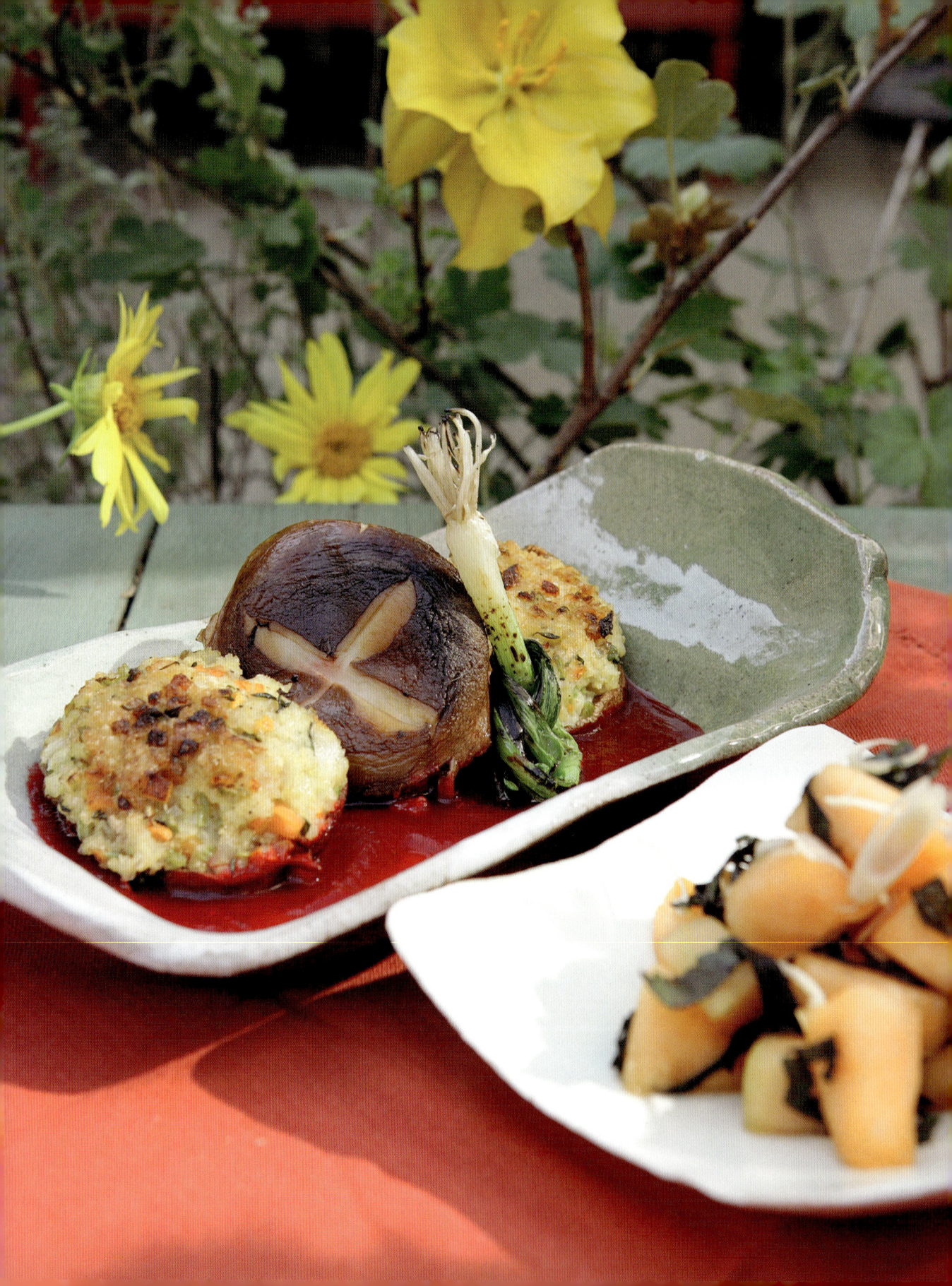

Stuffed Shiitake Mushrooms

with Millet and Kudzu Beet Sauce

Wow your guests with the elegance of this shiitake and millet dish. Mushroom lovers rejoice!

MAKES 4 SERVINGS

For the millet:
½ cup millet
1 ½ cups purified water
1 pinch sea salt

For the sauce:
½ onion, diced
¼ cup purified water, plus an additional 1 ½ cups water and 1 teaspoon water
1 red beet, diced
1 yellow beet, diced
1 tablespoon oregano, chopped
1 pinch sea salt
¼ teaspoon umeboshi vinegar
1 teaspoon kudzu

For the stuffed mushrooms:
2 tablespoons olive oil, divided
¼ cup onion, diced
¼ cup carrot, diced
¼ cup celery, diced
2 sprigs fresh thyme
1 pinch sea salt
10 to 12 fresh shiitake mushrooms, with 2- to 3-inch caps

To make the millet:
1. Pour the millet into a mesh strainer. Place strainer in a bowl under cold running water and rinse until the water is clear, usually three times or more. Drain thoroughly.
2. Transfer the grains to a medium saucepan. Over medium heat, parch the grains, stirring frequently, until dry.
3. Add the water and sea salt. Bring to a boil, cover and simmer for 20 minutes. Remove from heat, transfer to a large bowl, and allow to cool.

To make the sauce:
1. In a saucepan, combine the onions and ¼ cup of the water. "Water sauté"* until onions become translucent.
2. Add the beets, oregano, sea salt and water. Bring to a boil, lower the heat and simmer for 20 minutes or until beets are tender.
3. In a small bowl, dissolve the kudzu in a teaspoon of water.
4. Add the ume vinegar and kudzu to the pan and simmer for 2 minutes more. Transfer to a blender and purée until smooth. Set aside until ready to use.

To make the stuffed mushrooms:
1. In a wide saucepan, warm 1 tablespoon of the oil. Sauté the onions, carrot and celery for 2 minutes.
2. Add the thyme and sea salt and continue cooking for another minute. Transfer mixture to the bowl of millet and stir well to combine.
3. Stuff each shiitake with about 2 ounces of the millet mixture while still warm.
4. Warm the remaining tablespoon of the oil and panfry the stuffed shiitake, millet side down first, for a few minutes on each side.
5. Serve warm with the Kudzu Beet Sauce on the side.

*see page 31 for water sauté instructions

melon and thai basil pickles
with Lemongrass

This unique combination brings an equally unique taste that will satisfy your palate!

MAKES 4 SERVINGS

For the pickles:

1 cantaloupe melon (not overripe), diced
10 leaves thai basil, coarsely chopped
2-inch piece of lemongrass, very thinly sliced
1 teaspoon sea salt

To make the pickles:

1. In a large bowl, combine the melon and basil.
2. Add the lemongrass and sea salt, and mix well.
3. Transfer to a pickle press* and apply moderate pressure for 1 hour.
4. Remove pickles from press and rinse if they taste too salty. Drain off excess liquid and serve. Pickles will keep for up to 3 days in the refrigerator.

*see equipment list on page 90

ORGANIC Baby Yellow Wax Beans $4.75 lb.

ORGANIC Cantelope Melons $1.30 lb.

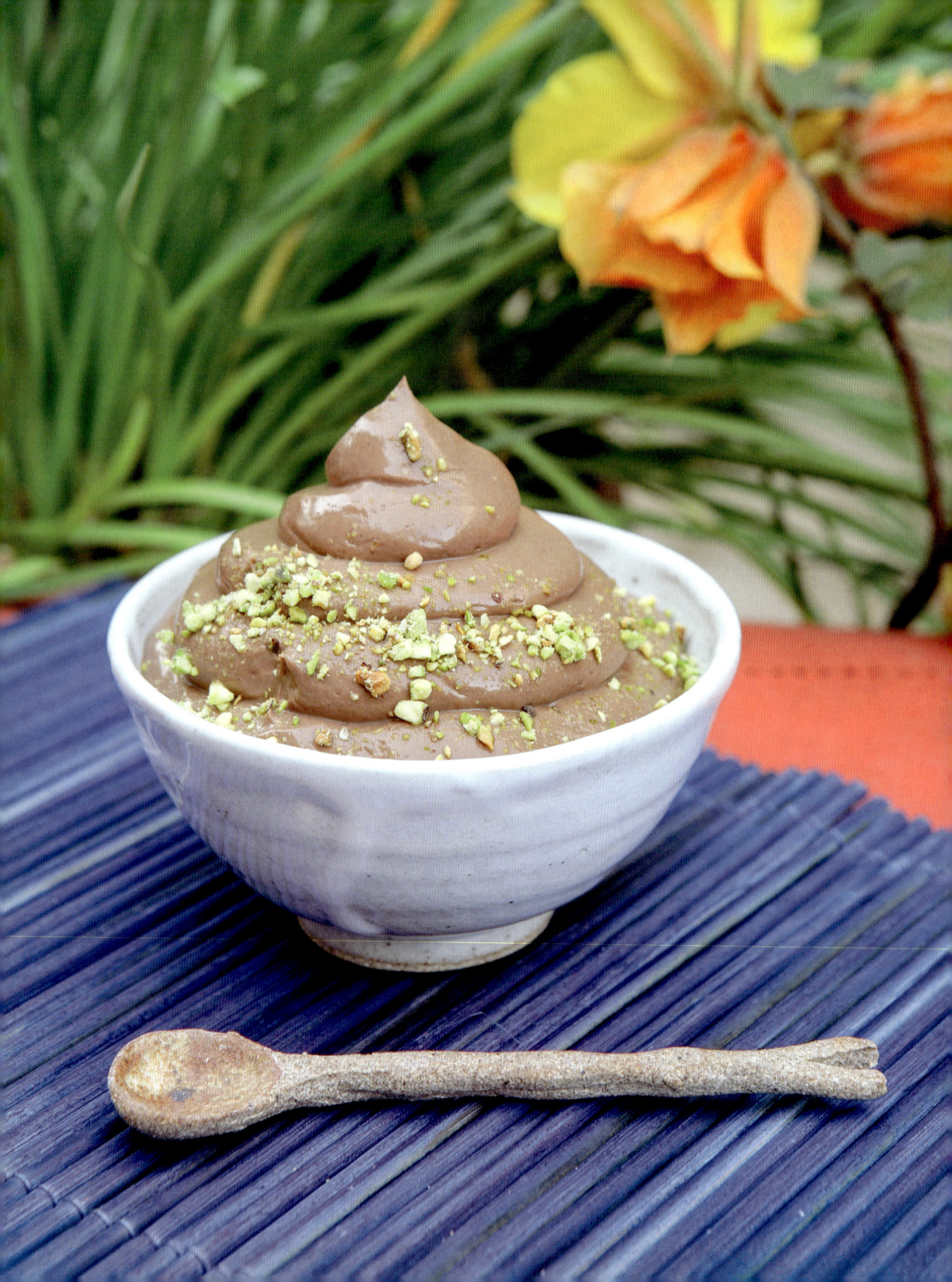

pistachio chocolate mousse

Chocolate lovers' heaven!

MAKES 4 TO 6 SERVINGS

For the mousse:
24 ounces silken firm tofu, well drained
½ cup maple sugar
1 pinch sea salt
½ cup soy milk (unsweetened)
9 ounces grain-sweetened chocolate chips
1 tablespoon vanilla extract
½ cup ground pistachios, divided

To make the mousse:
1. In a food processor, combine the tofu, maple sugar and sea salt, and process until very creamy, about 5 minutes.
2. In a saucepan over medium heat, combine the soy milk and chocolate chips. Stir continuously until chocolate has melted. Transfer to the food processor containing the tofu mixture.
3. Add the vanilla extract and process for a few more minutes.
4. Add ¼ cup of the pistachios and process until well combined.
5. Transfer mixture to a container and refrigerate for a few hours until well chilled.
6. Serve in individual bowls, garnished with the remaining pistachios.

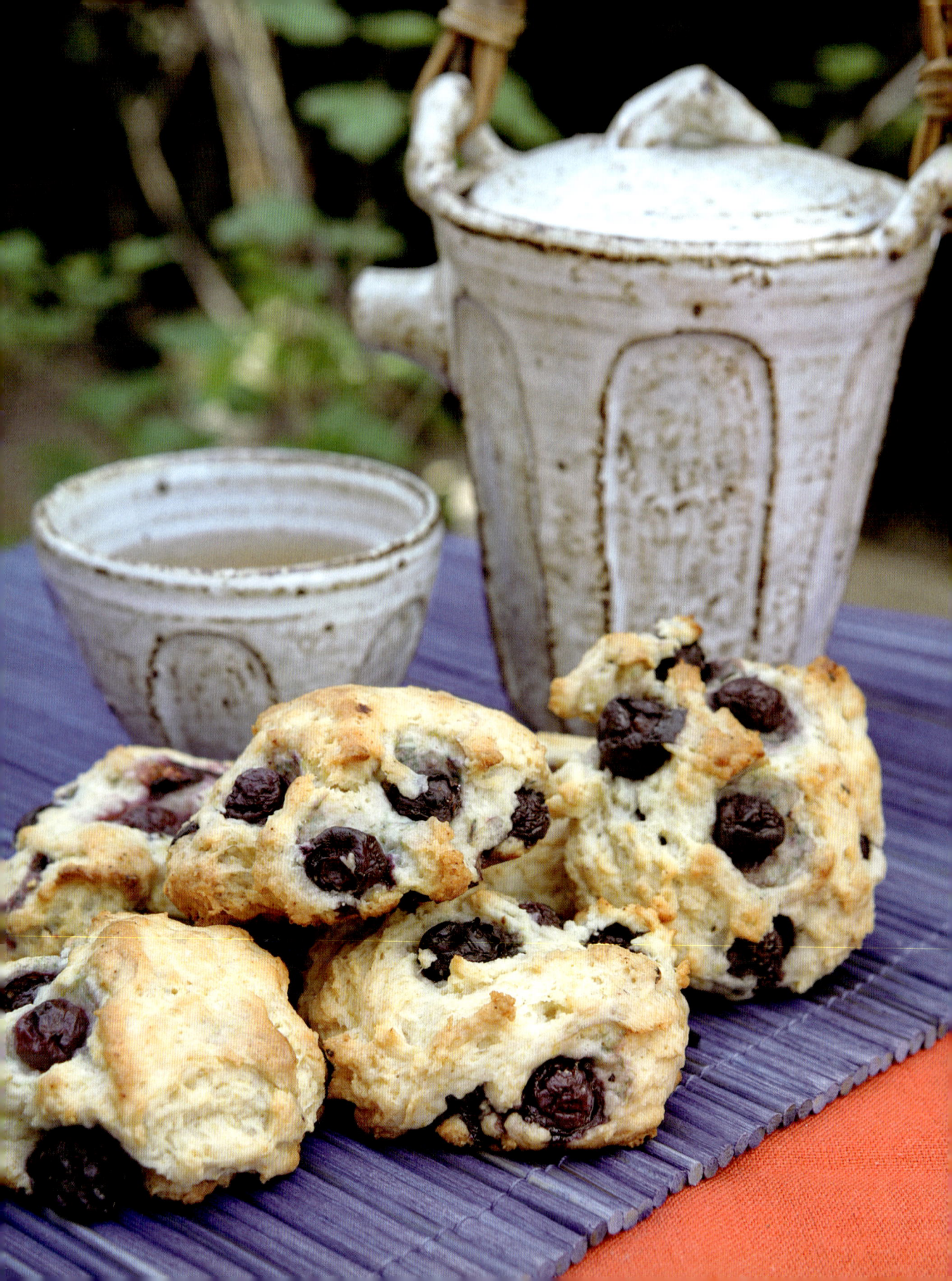

mini blueberry scones

Just before blueberry season is over, make lots of scones and indulge your loved ones.

MAKES 24 MINI SCONES

For the scones:
8 ounces silken firm tofu
1 cup safflower oil
¼ cup apple juice
¾ cup maple syrup
2 cups organic unbleached flour
2 cups organic whole wheat pastry flour
2 tablespoons baking powder
1 pinch sea salt
10 ounces blueberries

To make the scones:
1. Preheat the oven to 350°F.
2. In a blender, purée the tofu with the oil, apple juice and maple syrup.
3. Sift together the flour, baking powder and sea salt.
4. Combine the tofu mixture with the flour and fold by hand until the dough is soft but not sticky.
5. Add the blueberries to the dough and knead gently.
6. Using a 2-ounce ice cream scoop, drop dough 2 inches apart on a baking pan lined with parchment paper.
7. Bake for 25 to 30 minutes, or until golden brown.

Kukicha
with Rose Hips and Petals

Sometimes just plain Kukicha is not enough, don't you agree? So toss in a few rose hips and petals for a new taste and a dose of Vitamin C.

MAKES 2 SERVINGS

For the tea:
4 teaspoons Kukicha (Twig Tea)
2 teaspoons rose hips and petals
2 cups purified water

To make the tea:
1. Bring water to a boil. Combine the twigs, rose hips and petals in a teapot.
2. Pour the water over the tea and allow to steep for 5 minutes.
3. Strain and drink hot.

In autumn, look up at the sky. The sun is so far away—it felt as if it was within our reach in summer. Although we miss the sun, time seems to slow down during autumn, giving us space for self-reflection in preparation for winter.

Take the time to be sensitive and feel the sadness and joy, as we remember the good things from the past. Make an inventory of your feelings. Breathe deeply through your chest. Relax into the comforting and receiving energy of the season.

autumn

Butternut Squash and Kidney Bean Potage

Root Vegetable Pot Pie

Breaded Rice Balls with Lotus Seed

Shredded Daikon Salad with Pink Peppercorns

Mihama Hijiki with Edamame and Roasted Pumpkin Seeds

Lotus Root Pickles

Persimmon and Watercress with Asian Pear

Black Sesame Dumplings with Warm Coconut Soup

Walnut Cookies

Genmaicha

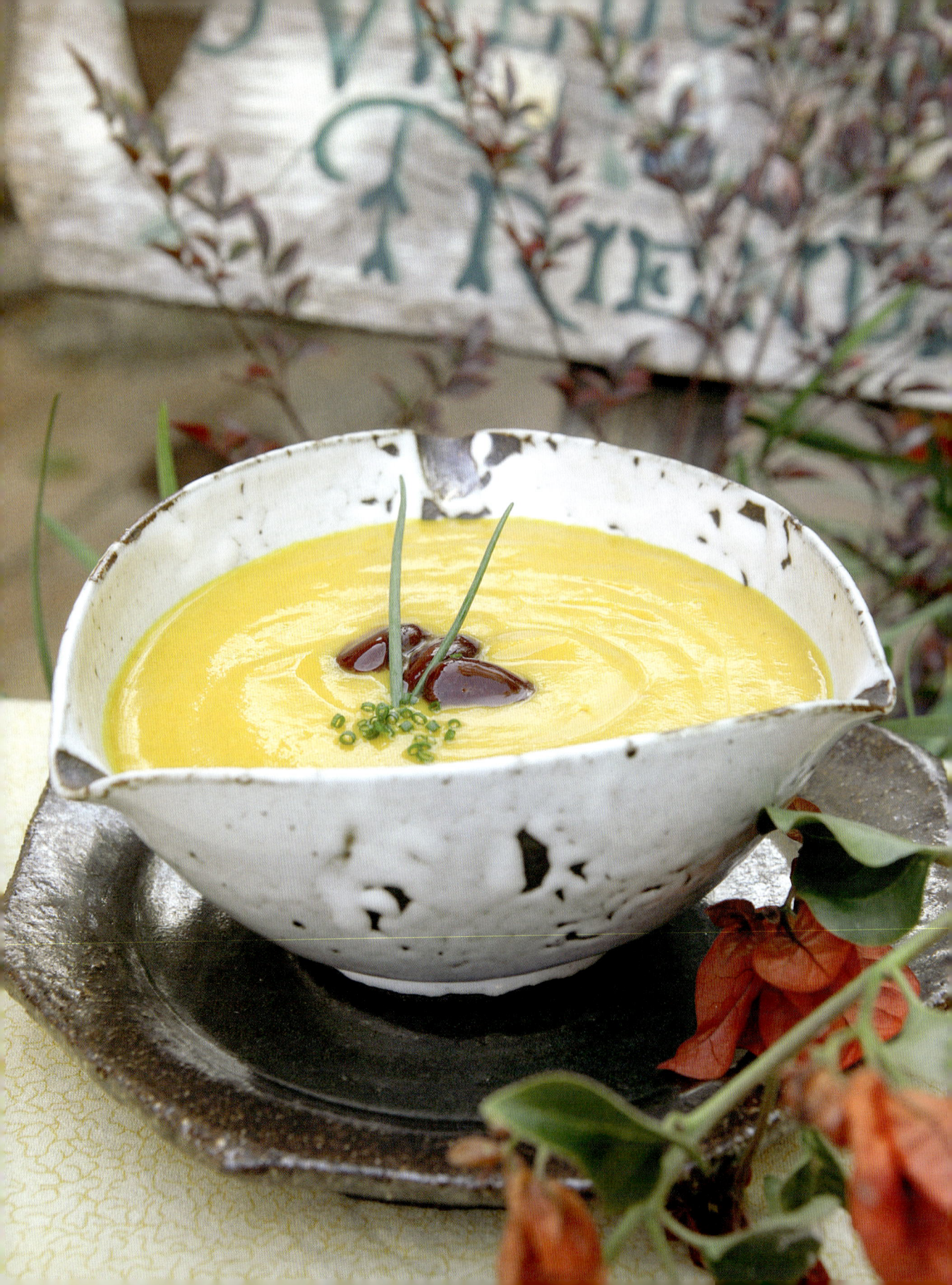

butternut squash and kidney bean potage

We wanted to make something special out of the common butternut squash soup by combining it with kidney beans. The result will surprise you.

MAKES 4 SERVINGS

For the kidney beans:
¼ cup kidney beans, sorted and rinsed
2 cups water
1-inch strip of kombu

For the squash soup:
1 butternut squash
2 tablespoons olive oil
1 brown onion, finely diced
2 carrots, finely diced
2 cups water
2 pinches sea salt
2 pinches curry powder
1 tablespoon white miso
½ cup rice milk (unsweetened)

To make the kidney beans:
1. Soak the beans in ample water for 4 to 6 hours. Drain.
2. In a large pot with a lid, combine the beans, water and kombu and bring to a boil.
3. Cover and simmer for 40 minutes, or until beans are fully cooked and still retain their shape.

To make the squash soup:
1. Using a vegetable peeler, peel the squash, slice in half, and remove the seeds. Coarsely chop the squash and set aside.
2. In a medium saucepan, warm the oil. Sauté the onions lightly for a few minutes.
3. Add the carrots, squash, and water, and simmer for a few minutes.
4. Add the sea salt and curry powder. Bring to a boil, reduce heat, and simmer for 20 minutes.
5. Transfer vegetables to a blender. Add the miso and rice milk and purée until creamy.
5. Transfer to a large bowl or pot, gently stir in the whole beans and serve.

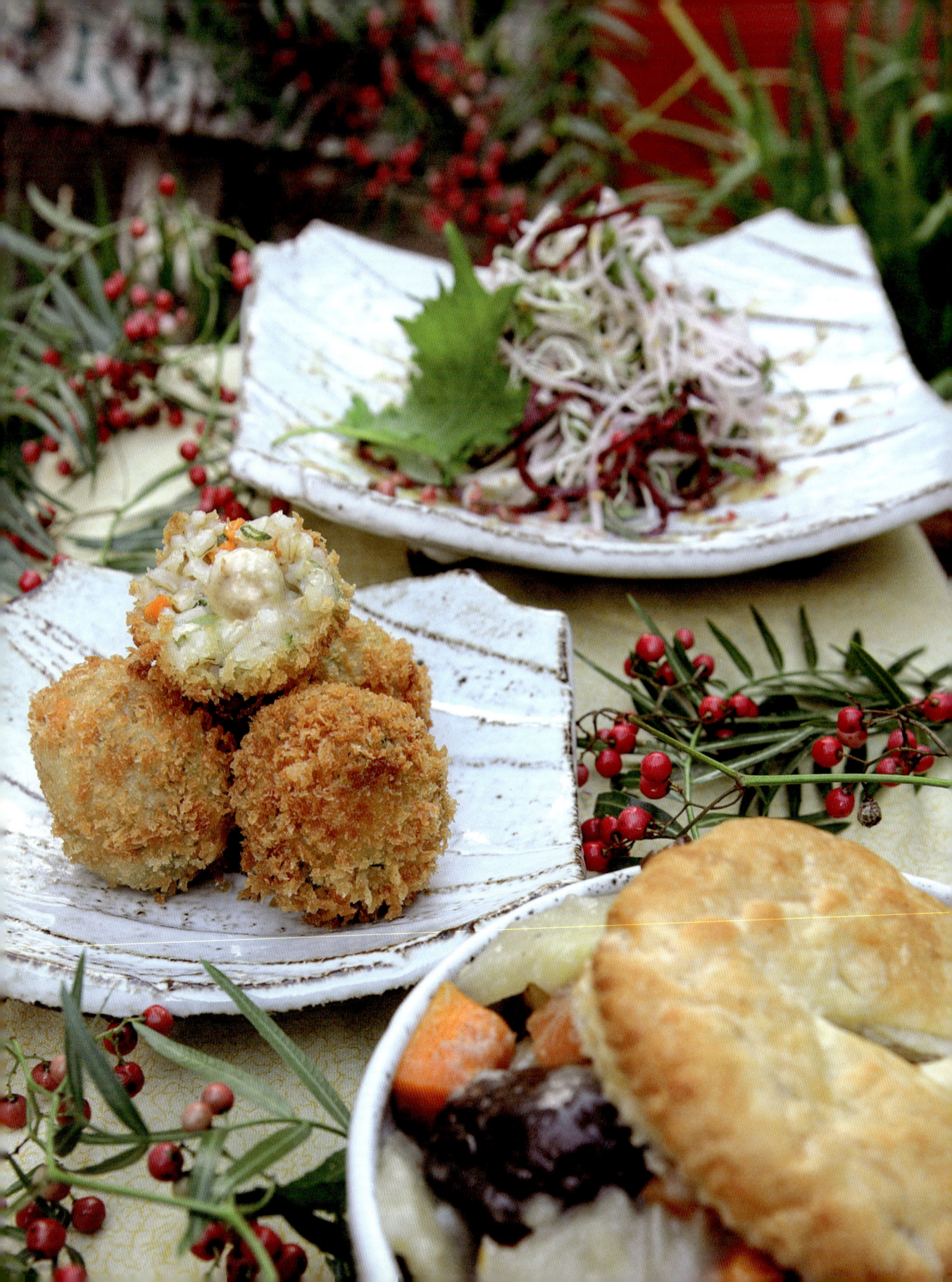

root vegetable pot pie

A great dish to introduce root vegetables to your guests who don't usually venture farther than potatoes.

MAKES 4 SERVINGS

For the puff pastry:
- 1 cup unbleached flour
- ½ cup whole wheat pastry flour
- 5 ounces soy margarine, chilled
- 2 teaspoons white wine vinegar, chilled
- 3 ⅓ to 4 ⅔ tablespoons water, chilled

For the vegetables:
- 1 tablespoon sesame oil
- 3 shiitake mushrooms, quartered
- ½ cup parsnips, cubed
- ½ cup jinenjo root
- ½ onion, cubed
- ½ carrot, cubed
- 1 pinch thyme
- 1 pinch herb de provence
- 1 pinch sea salt
- 1 cup kombu dashi (recipe on page 15)
- 1 tablespoon kudzu
- ¼ cup soy milk (unsweetened)

To make the puff pastry:
1. In a food processor, combine the soy margarine and flours. Process until the mixture resembles a coarse meal, about 10 seconds.
2. Add vinegar and 3 ⅓ tablespoons of the chilled water, and pulse for 5 to 6 seconds. Scrape down the mixture and pulse for another 3 to 4 seconds. The dough should just hold together. If the mixture is still crumbly, add more chilled water and pulse for 2 to 3 seconds more.
3. On a lightly floured surface, use a rolling pin to roll the dough away from you into a rectangle.
4. Fold the ends closest and furthest from you to the center. Then fold in half, like closing a book, to create 4 layers.
5. Turn 90° and repeat steps 3 and 4.
6. Refrigerate for 10 minutes and then repeat steps 3, 4 and 5 two more times.
7. Keep refrigerated until ready to use.

To make the vegetables and assemble the pot pie:
1. Preheat the oven to 325° F.
2. In a large pan, warm the oil. Sauté the vegetables for 3 to 4 minutes.
3. Add the herbs, salt and kombu dashi and bring to a boil. Cover and simmer for about 10 minutes, until the vegetables are tender.
4. In a small bowl, dissolve the kudzu in the soy milk. Add to the vegetables and stir well with a wooden spoon. The mixture will become thick and creamy. Transfer to an 8-inch baking pan (or four 4-inch ramekins).
5. Roll the dough out to a ¼-inch thickness and transfer to cover the top of the pan (or each ramekin).
6. Trim excess dough around the edges and bake for 15 minutes or until golden.

breaded rice balls
with Lotus Seeds

Lotus seeds have excellent healing properties. These rice balls are great for snacks, party trays, or when you just need something to "hit the spot."

MAKES 4 SERVINGS

For the rice balls:
2 cups brown rice, short grain
¼ cup lotus seeds, soaked
3 cups purified water
1 pinch sea salt
1 tablespoon sesame oil
¼ cup carrot, diced
¼ cup celery, diced
¼ cup scallions, diced

For the breading:
1 cup soy milk (unsweetened)
1 tablespoon mustard
1 cup whole grain flour
1 cup sourdough bread crumbs
safflower oil (for deep frying)

To make the rice balls:
1. Add the rice to a mesh strainer. Place strainer in a bowl under cold running water and rinse until the water is clear, usually three times or more. Drain thoroughly.
2. Transfer the rice to a pressure cooker. Add the lotus seeds, water and sea salt.
3. Bring up to pressure, and simmer for 50 minutes.
4. Meanwhile, in a medium sauté pan warm the oil over a medium flame. Add the carrots, celery and scallions and gently cook for a few minutes. Set aside.
5. When the rice is ready, stir and fluff the grains gently with a wet, wooden spatula or spoon.
6. Stir in the cooked vegetables.
7. Using a moistened 1-ounce ice cream scoop, form the rice mixture into balls. Set aside on a platter.

To bread the rice balls:
1. In a small mixing bowl, combine the milk and mustard.
2. In two separate mixing bowls, place the flour by itself in one, and the bread crumbs by itself in the other.
3. Dip a rice ball in the flour, then the soy milk mixture, then the bread crumbs and transfer back to the platter.
4. Repeat with remaining rice balls.
5. Deep fry the breaded rice balls in oil (2 to 3 inches deep) at 325°F until golden brown. Drain on paper towels and serve immediately.

Shredded daikon salad
with Pink Peppercorns

In autumn, we love to go hiking and have fun picking wild pink peppercorns. They add a pleasant bite to this simple yet refreshing salad.

MAKES 4 SERVINGS

For the dressing:
2 tablespoons grain mustard
1 tablespoon brown rice vinegar
1 pinch sea salt
freshly cracked pepper
¼ cup olive oil or sesame oil

For the salad:
1 daikon, 10- to 12-inches long
1 tablespoon pink peppercorns, crushed
1 bunch Shiso leaves, about 6 to 8 leaves
1 red beet, thinly sliced
1 package alfalfa sprouts

To make the dressing:
1. In a small bowl, combine the mustard, vinegar, salt and pepper.
2. Whisk in the oil gently, until well blended.
3. Transfer to a container and refrigerate.

To make the salad:
1. Using a vegetable slicer, shred the daikon, spaghetti-style.
2. Bring a large pot of water to a boil and quickly blanch the daikon, plunge in ice water and drain. Transfer daikon to dry between 2 towels.
3. Thinly slice the shiso leaves.
4. In a large serving bowl, combine the daikon, shiso, beets, alfalfa, and peppercorns. Toss with the dressing just before serving.

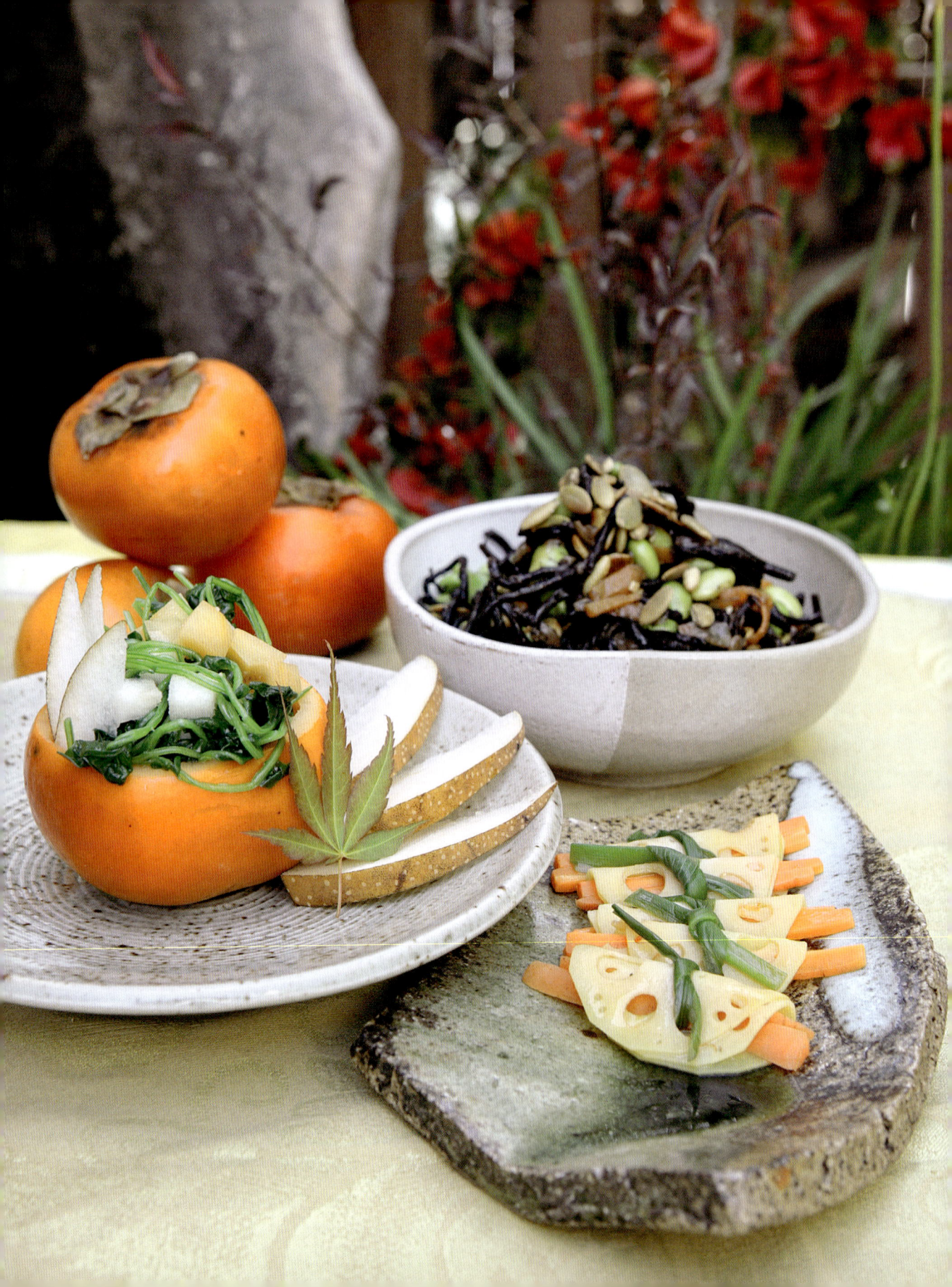

AUTUMN — LOVE, ERIC & SANAE

mihama hijiki
with Edamame and Roasted Pumpkin Seeds

Sea vegetables are a great source of calcium, especially hijiki. Combined with edamame protein, this is a powerhouse dish. The hijiki pictured is a very thick and long variety that comes from the Japanese village of Mihama (Sanae's mother's hometown).

MAKES 4 SERVINGS

For the hijiki:
2 ounces hijiki
1 cup of purified water
2 tablespoons sesame oil
½ brown onion, sliced
2 tablespoons mirin (optional)
1 carrot, shredded
2 tablespoons soy sauce
1 cup edamame
1 cup roasted pumpkin seeds

To make the hijiki:
1. Rinse the hijiki and soak for 10 minutes. Reserve soaking water.
2. In a large pan, warm the oil. Sauté the onions for about 2 minutes.
3. Add mirin and cook for another minute.
4. Add the hijiki and carrot to the pan, along with ½ of the hijiki-soaking water. Bring to a boil, cover, and simmer for 20 minutes.
5. Add soy sauce and continue cooking for a few more minutes.
6. Remove from heat and stir in the edamame.
7. Allow to cool and serve garnished with pumpkin seeds.

lotus root pickles

Lotus root is a very attractive vegetable. We think this artistic dish will be one of your favorites.

MAKES 4 SERVINGS

For the pickles:
1 lotus root, about 5 inches long, thinly sliced
1 carrot, cut into sticks (about 3 inches long and ¼-inch thick)
1 pinch saffron
6 tablespoons rice vinegar
1 teaspoon sea salt
3 scallions, white part removed

To make the pickles:
1. In a large saucepan, combine the lotus root, carrots, saffron, vinegar and sea salt.
2. Bring to a boil, cover, and simmer for 10 minutes. Allow to cool and set aside.
3. Bring a pot of water to boil. Blanch the whole scallions, plunge in ice water, and drain.
4. Wrap a few carrot pieces between 2 slices of lotus root (like a taco) and tie closed with a strand of scallion.
5. Will stay fresh for a few days within a sealed container in the refrigerator.

persimmon and watercress
with Asian Pear

One of the fruit trees in our garden is a glorious persimmon. In this dish, the colors of autumn harmonize with contrasting flavors, and become a delicious and decorative masterpiece.

MAKES 4 SERVINGS

For the ginger dressing:
1 tablespoon white miso
½ tablespoon ginger juice
1 tablespoon rice vinegar
3 tablespoons safflower oil or sesame oil

For the salad:
1 bunch watercress
4 persimmons
1 asian pear, sliced

To make the ginger dressing:
1. In a small bowl, combine the miso, ginger juice, and rice vinegar.
2. Whisk in the oil gently and set aside.

To make the salad:
1. Bring a pot of water to a boil. Quickly blanch the watercress, plunge in ice water, and drain.
2. Coarsely chop the watercress and set aside.
3. Slice the top off of each persimmon and scoop out the inside flesh. Keep the persimmon "cup" and dice the scooped-out fruit.
4. In a large bowl, combine the watercress, diced persimmons, and sliced pear. Pour the dressing over the salad and toss to coat.
5. Transfer the salad into each persimmon cup and serve.

AUTUMN — LOVE, ERIC & SANAE

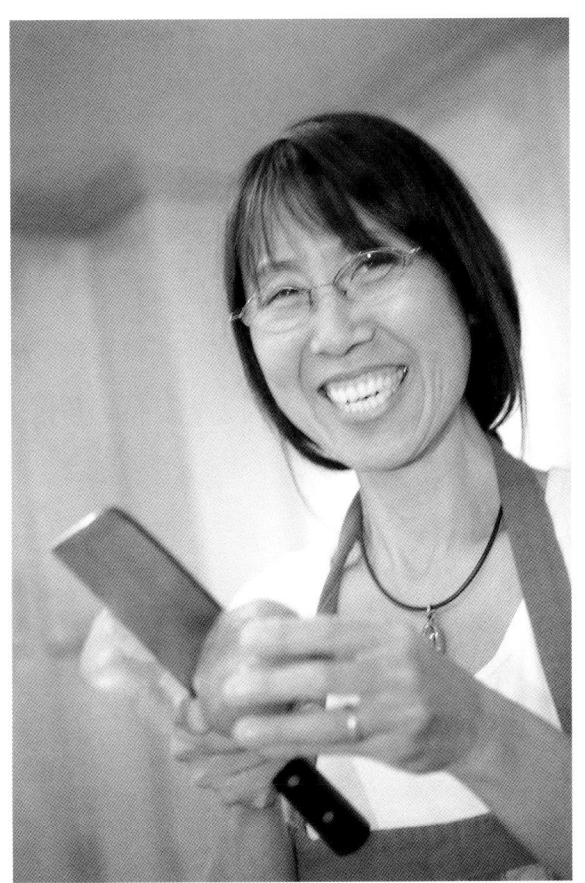
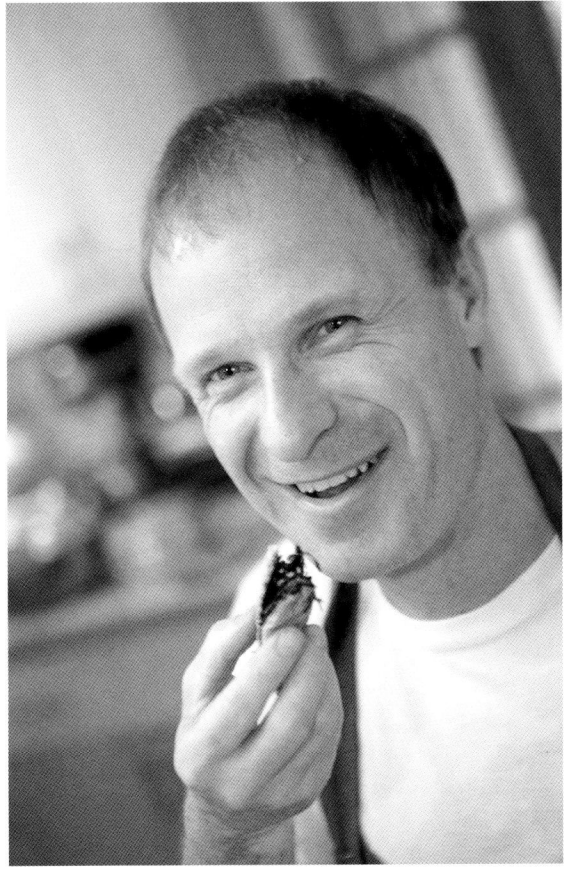

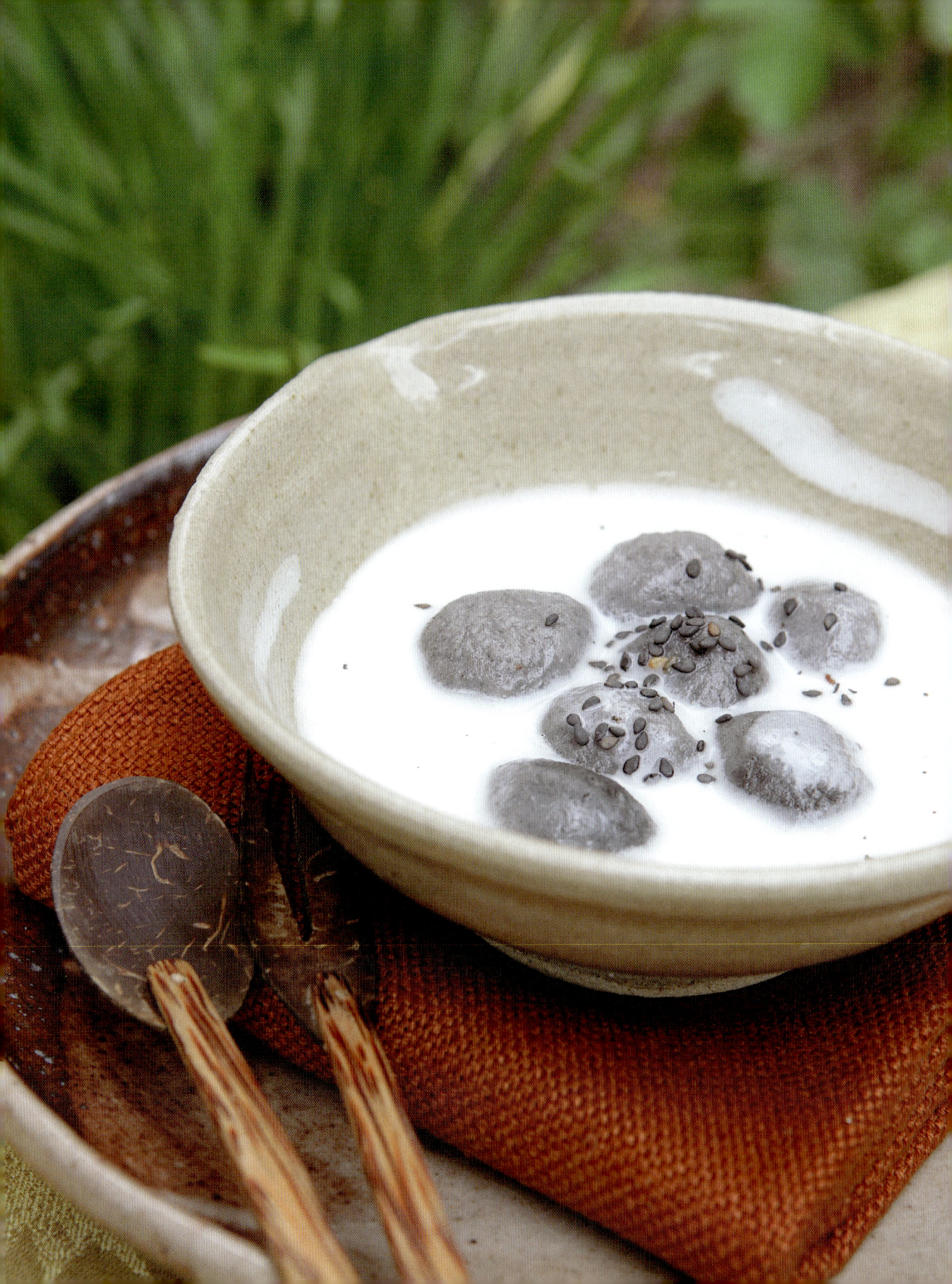

black sesame dumplings
with Warm Coconut Soup

The inspiration for this recipe came to us during our travels to Beijing, China. It's a truly delectable dessert!

MAKES 4 SERVINGS

For the dumplings:
½ cup sweet rice flour
½ cup water
1 tablespoon black sesame paste
1 pinch sea salt

For the soup:
1 can organic coconut milk
1 tablespoon rice syrup
1 vanilla bean

Optional garnish:
black sesame seeds, roasted

To make the dumplings:
1. In a small mixing bowl, combine the flour, water, black sesame paste and sea salt.
2. With wet hands, form 14 to 16 balls from the flour mixture, about ¼-ounce each.
3. Fill a large pot of water halfway full. Add the sea salt and bring to a boil.
4. Drop the dumplings in the boiling water and cook for about 2 minutes after they come up to the surface.
5. Drain, plunge in cold water and allow to cool.

To make the soup:
1. In a medium saucepan, combine the coconut milk and rice syrup.
2. Split the vanilla bean and add it to the milk. Simmer for a few minutes.
3. Remove the bean with a slotted spoon, scrape out the seeds, and transfer the seeds back into the pan. Stir to combine.
4. Divide the milk and dumplings among 4 soup bowls and serve garnished with sesame seeds.

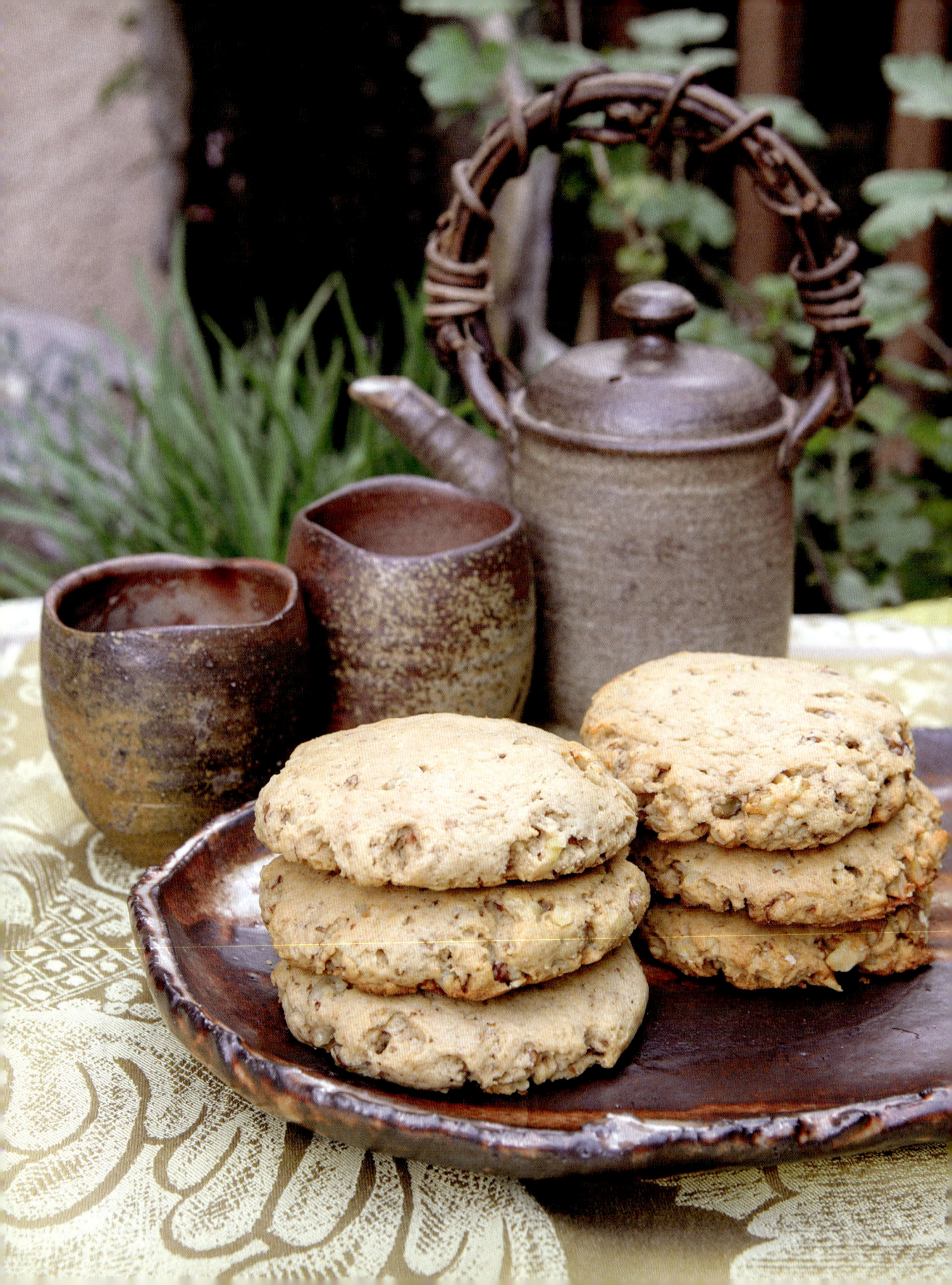

walnut cookies

One of our favorites... actually Sanae's absolute favorite!

MAKES 12 SERVINGS

For the cookies:
4 ounces silken firm tofu
8 ounces soy margarine
   (or 4 ounces safflower oil
   plus 1 pinch sea salt)
2 cups unbleached flour
¼ cup whole wheat pastry flour
¼ teaspoon baking powder
¼ teaspoon baking soda
2 ounces maple sugar
6 ounces walnuts, chopped
¼ cup brown rice syrup
2 teaspoons vanilla extract

To make the cookies:
1. Preheat the oven to 350° F.
2. In a food processor, process the tofu until creamy. Add the margarine or safflower oil. If using oil, add the pinch of salt. Pulse for 2 to 3 seconds.
3. In a large bowl, combine the flours, baking soda, baking powder, maple sugar, and walnuts.
4. Add the tofu mixture, rice syrup, and vanilla extract to the dry ingredients, and stir together by hand.
5. Using a 2-ounce ice cream scoop, drop cookie dough about 2 inches apart onto a baking pan lined with parchment paper.
6. Bake for 12 to 15 minutes, until golden brown.

genmaicha
Roasted Brown Rice Tea

Brown rice is harvested in autumn. Roast your own brown rice for a hearty cup of Genmaicha and celebrate this season.

MAKES 2 SERVINGS

For the tea:
2 tablespoons Genmaicha*
2 cups purified water

To make the tea:
1. Bring water to a boil. Add the tea to a teapot.
2. Pour the water over the tea and allow to steep for 5 minutes.
3. Strain and drink hot.

*To make your own genmaicha:
In a skillet, roast 1 tablespoon of brown rice until grains puff up. Combine rice with 2 tablespoons of kukicha.

This is the season of hope. Even though the cold season depresses us, if we remember to relax and practice our patience, we know that the beautiful season of spring is approaching.

Winter is a difficult time, and we often feel fear, and worry about everything and anything. In light of this, the best plan is to keep ourselves warm, and to spend time with our families, friends and pets, remembering to tell them how much we love them. Love will cure everything!

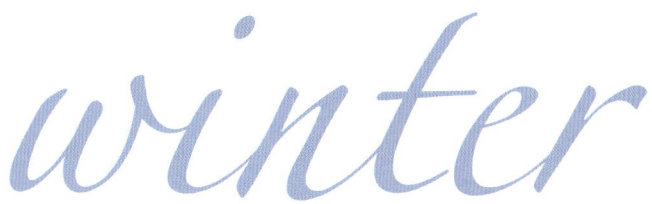

winter

French Onion Soup with Crispy Mochi

Seitan Bourguignon

Buckwheat and Brown Rice

Red Radish and Green Top Pickles

Krispy Kombu Chips

Savoy Cabbage with Walnut and Carrot Sauce

Braised Whole Burdock

Apple Cinnamon Strudel

Oatmeal Cherry Kisses

Soy Latte Grain Coffee

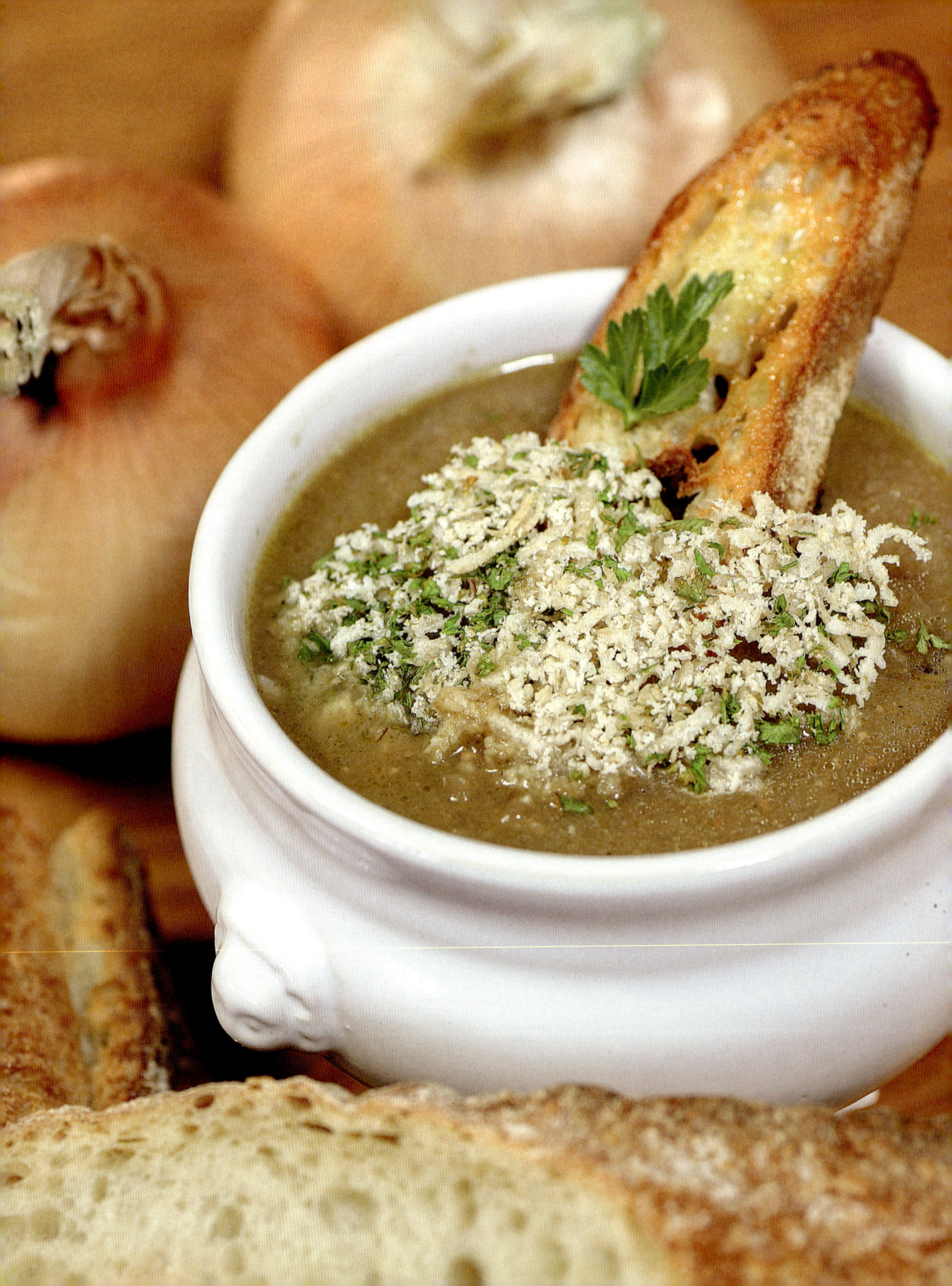

French Onion Soup
with Crispy Mochi

Onion soup without cheese? No problem. Not only will you be fully satisfied, but you'll love it!

MAKES 4 SERVINGS

For the mochi:
8 tablespoons plain mochi, grated

For the soup:
3 tablespoons olive oil or sesame oil
2 brown onions, thinly sliced
2 pinches sea salt
2 tablespoons spelt flour
4 cups kombu dashi (recipe on page 15)
2 bay leaves
1 tablespoon fresh thyme, chopped
1 tablespoon white miso
1 tablespoon country barley miso
8 pieces sourdough croutons
¼ cup plain mochi, grated

To make the mochi:
1. In a sauté pan over a medium-high flame, sprinkle 2 tablespoons grated mochi in a 3-inch circle. The mochi will melt together slightly and hold the circular shape.
2. Cook each side for 1 minute. Set aside and repeat for the others.

To make the soup:
1. In a large saucepan over a medium-high flame, warm the oil. Sauté the onions and sea salt until a golden brown color, about 12 to 15 minutes. Don't let the onion burn.
2. Add the spelt flour and mix well with a wooden spoon.
3. Add the kombu dashi one cup at a time and stir well. Bring to a boil, reduce heat, and simmer.
4. Add the bay leaves and thyme, and continue cooking for 50 to 60 minutes, stirring occasionally.
5. Stir in the miso and ¼ cup mochi. Keep stirring until well combined and cook for a few minutes more.
6. Pour soup into individual bowls, add sourdough croutons, and garnish with crispy mochi.
7. Serve while it's hot.

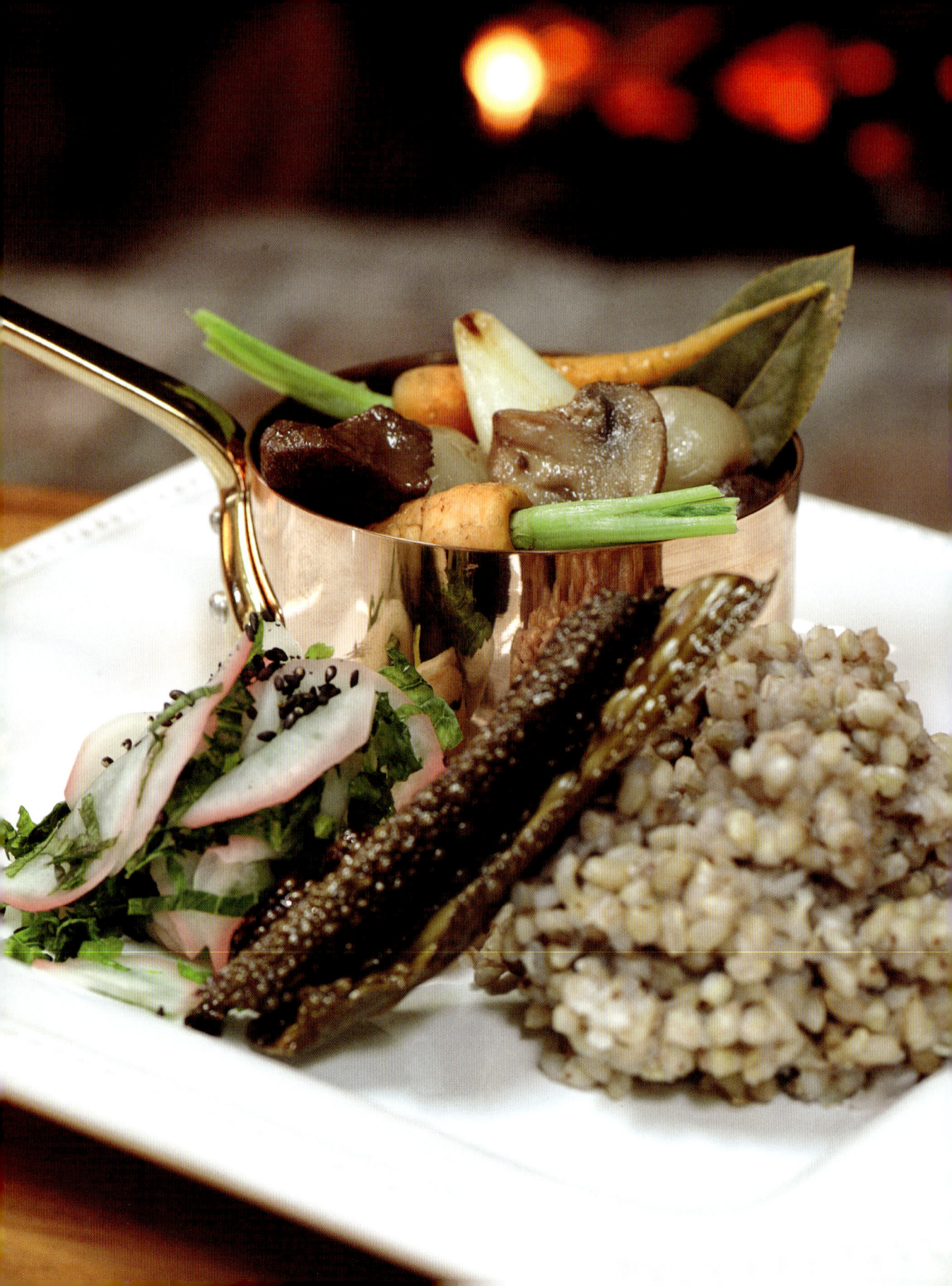

Seitan bourguignon

We love this stew during the cold winter season... it's Eric's favorite!

MAKES 4 SERVINGS

For the bourguignon:
1 ½ tablespoons olive oil or sesame oil
5 ounces pearl onions
1 bunch baby carrots or 2 carrots, diced
2 pinches sea salt
4 ounces button mushrooms
8 ounces seitan, cut into 1-inch cubes
1 ½ tablespoons spelt flour
¼ cup red wine (if desired)
1 ½ cups kombu dashi (recipe on page 15)
2 bay leaves
1 tablespoon soy sauce

To make bourguignon:
1. In a large saucepan, warm the oil. Sauté the pearl onions, carrots, and sea salt for a few minutes.
2. Add the mushrooms and seitan, and sauté for another minute.
3. Using a wooden spoon, add the spelt flour and stir well to combine.
4. Add the red wine and stir again.
5. Add the bay leaves and pour the kombu dashi over the mixture.
6. Bring to a boil, reduce heat, cover, and simmer for 30 minutes.
7. Season with soy sauce and serve.

buckwheat and brown rice

Buckwheat has a very nutty flavor that works well with brown rice.

MAKES 4 SERVINGS

For the grains:
1 cup buckwheat
1 cup brown rice
3 cups purified water
1 pinch sea salt

To make the grains:
1. Add the buckwheat to a mesh strainer. Place strainer in a bowl under cold running water and rinse until the water is clear, usually three times or more. Drain thoroughly and set aside. Repeat process with the brown rice. Transfer the brown rice to a large saucepan with a lid, add the purified water and soak for 4 to 6 hours.
2. Add the buckwheat and pinch of sea salt to the pan. Bring to a boil, cover and simmer for 50 minutes. Remove from heat and allow pan to sit for 5 to 10 minutes.

red radish and green top pickles

Pickles are so refreshing, but also a very important digestive aid.

MAKES 4 SERVINGS

For the pickles:
½ cup radish greens, chopped
½ cup red radishes, thinly sliced
½ teaspoon sea salt
¼ teaspoon black sesame seeds, roasted

To make the pickles:
1. In a large bowl, combine the greens, radish slices and sea salt.
2. Transfer to a pickle press*, apply pressure and let sit on a counter 2 to 3 hours.
3. Rinse pickles if they taste too salty. Squeeze out excess liquid by hand. Pickles will keep for up to 3 days in the refrigerator.
4. Serve with roasted sesame seeds as a garnish.

*see equipment list on page 90

crispy kombu chips

Wow, these are so good... you must make this, either as a snack or a side dish and try not to eat too much!

MAKES 4 SERVINGS

For the chips:
4 pieces of 4-inch strips of kombu
safflower oil, for deep frying

To make chips:
1. Wipe the kombu on both sides with a dry cloth.
2. In a skillet over medium-high heat, warm the oil (about 1 to 2 inches deep) to 350° F.
3. Fry the kombu on both sides until crispy and drain on paper towels.

WINTER — LOVE, ERIC & SANAE

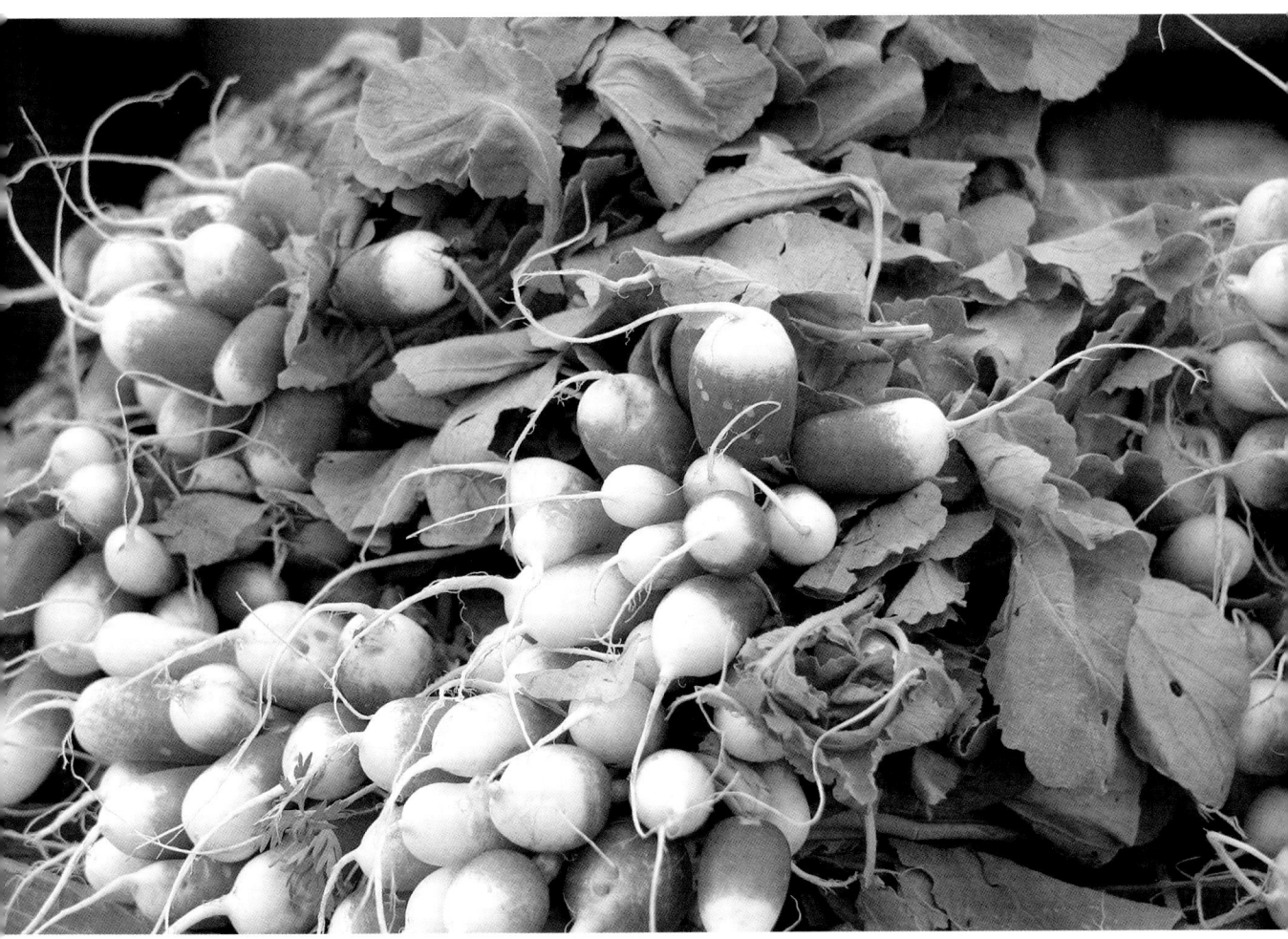

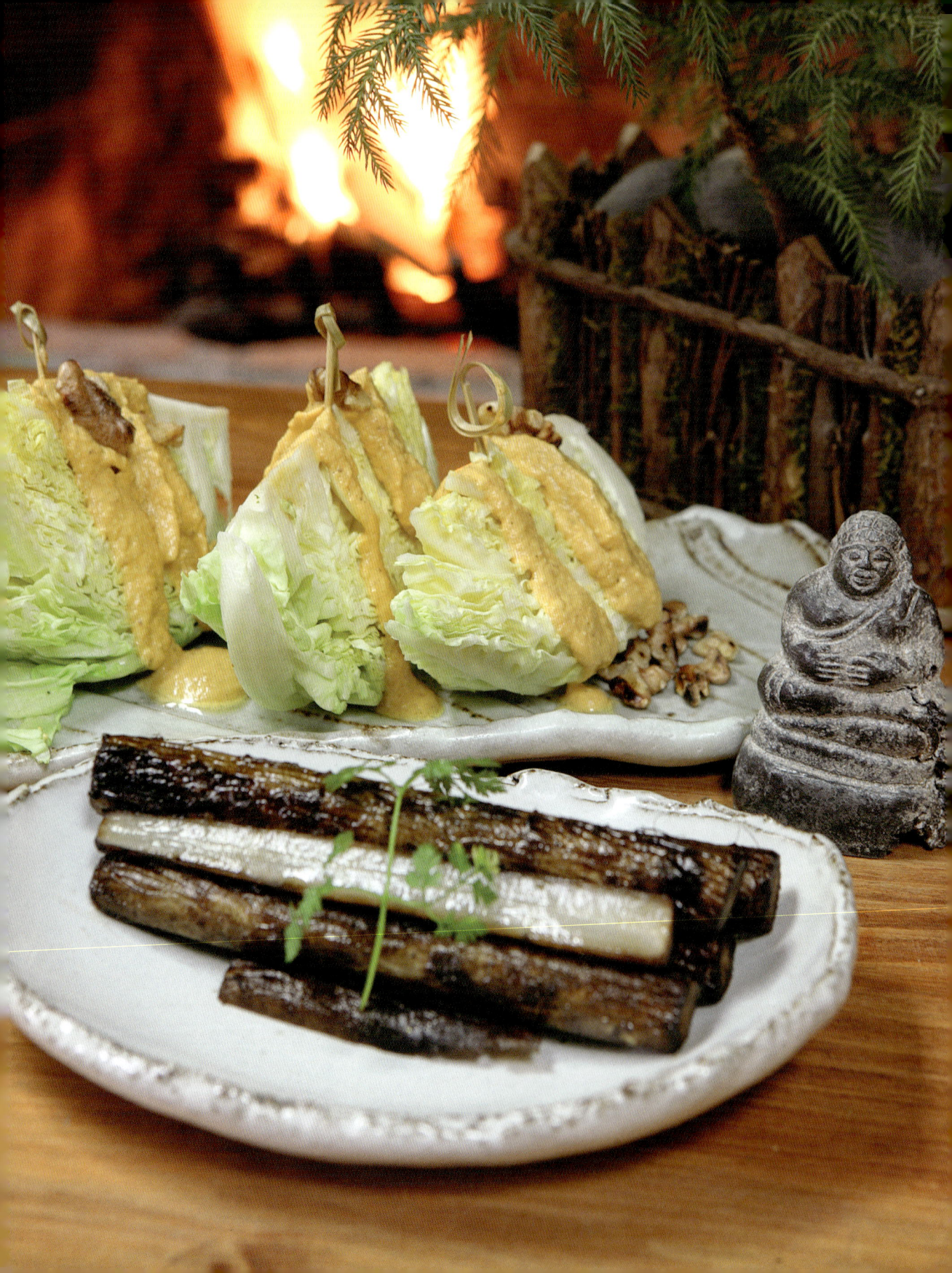

Savoy Cabbage
with Walnut and Carrot Sauce

We know winter is officially here when we see Savoy cabbage at our local farmer's market. The walnut sauce lends a rich creamy taste.

MAKES 4 SERVINGS

1 whole Savoy cabbage

For the cabbage:
1 whole Savoy cabbage

For the sauce:
1 cup roasted walnuts
2 carrots, diced, steamed and puréed
¾ cup kombu dashi (recipe on page 15)

To make the cabbage:
1. Slice the cabbage into 8 to 10 wedges from top to bottom.
2. In a pot fitted with a steamer, steam cabbage for 6 to 8 minutes, or until tender.

To make the sauce:
1. In a food processor or suribachi, purée the walnuts until creamy.
2. Add the carrot purée and kombu dashi and stir well to combine.
3. Season with sea salt, if needed.
4. Pour over the steamed cabbage wedges.

braised whole burdock

Burdock is a powerfully healing root vegetable, but better yet, this recipe is delightfully simple to prepare. Let it cook for a long time, then simply enjoy the goodness.

MAKES 4 SERVINGS

To make the burdock:
1 burdock root,
 about 15 to 20 inches long
1 tablespoon sesame oil
½ cup kombu dashi (recipe on page 15) or water
3 to 4 tablespoons soy sauce

Optional garnish:
a few sprigs of fresh chervil (as pictured)
or 1 tablespoon roasted sesame seeds

To make the burdock:
1. Scrub the burdock lightly using a natural fiber brush and slice into 5- to 6-inch logs.
2. In a large skillet over a medium-high flame, warm the oil. Panfry the burdock on all sides until crispy.
3. Add the dashi (or water) to cover the burdock. Bring to a boil, reduce heat to a medium flame, cover, and cook until the burdock is tender, adding additional water, if necessary.
4. Add the soy sauce and cook uncovered until almost all liquid has evaporated.
5. Allow to cool slightly, transfer to a serving dish and garnish with chervil or sesame seeds.

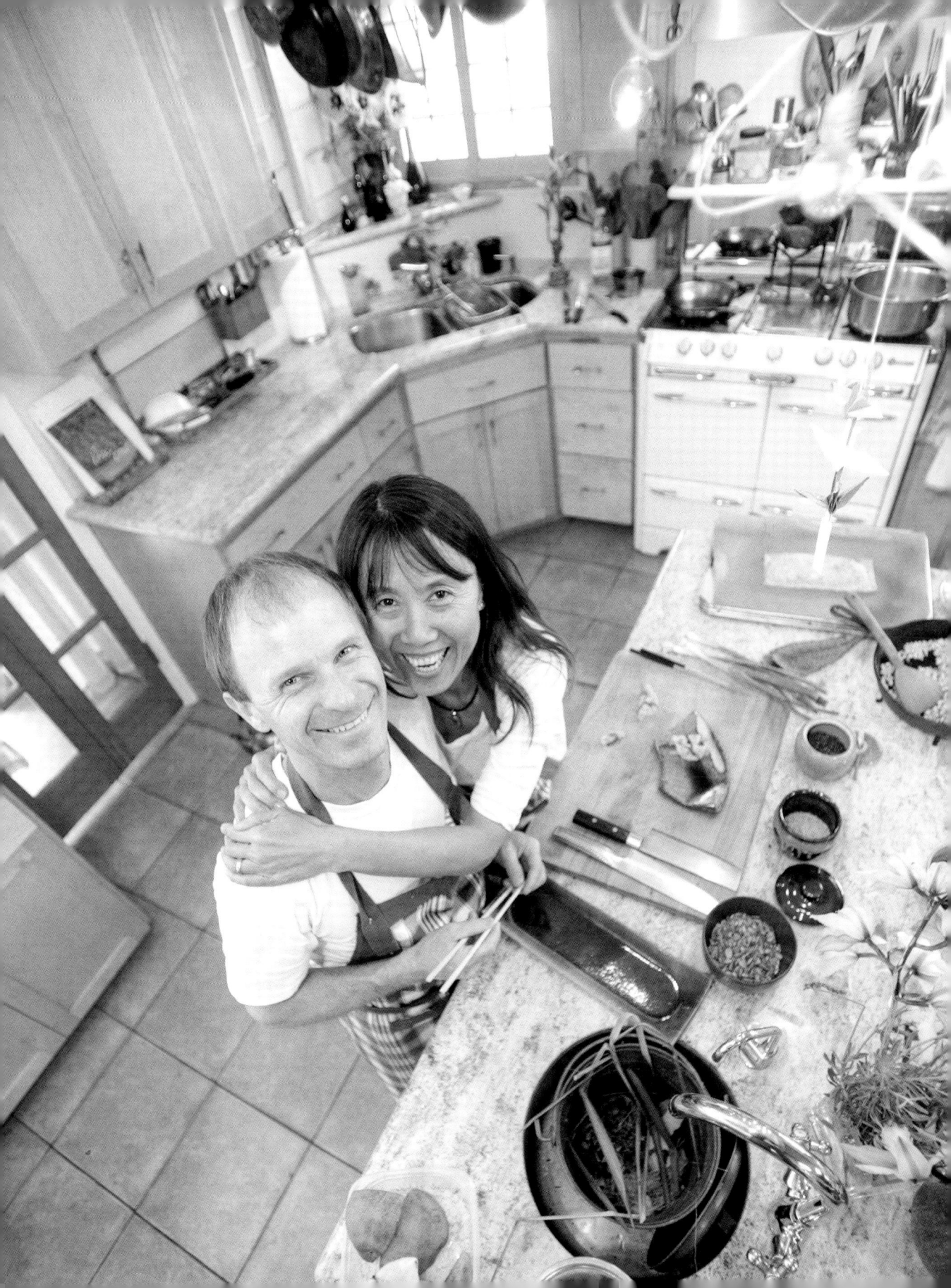

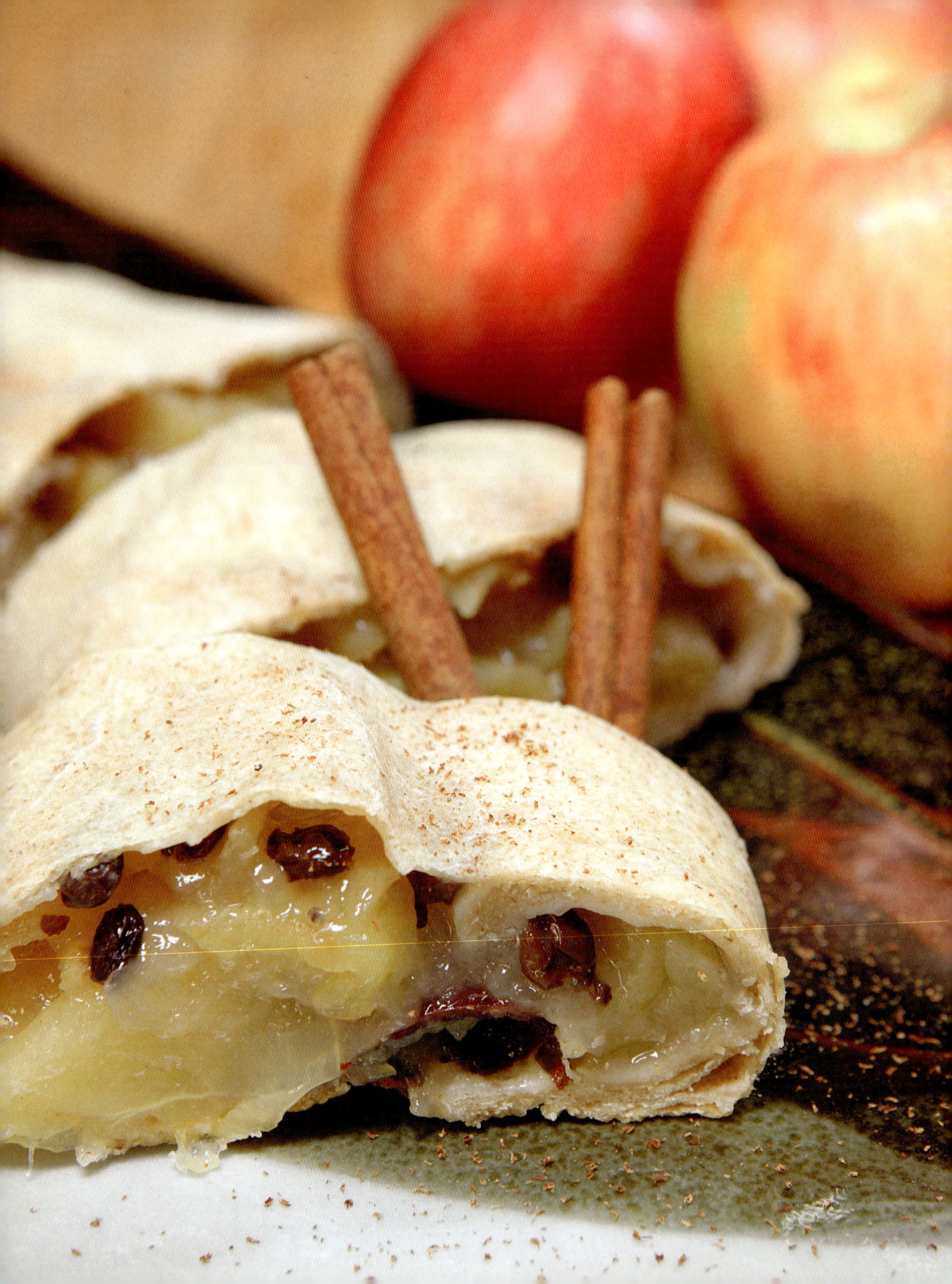

apple cinnamon strudel

This is a classic and still the best. Without butter this recipe is even more scrumptious, light, and easy on the heart.

MAKES 4 TO 6 SERVINGS

For the filling:
12 organic Fuji apples, peeled, cored and cut into ½-inch wedges
¾ cup brown rice syrup
3 cups organic apple juice
1 cinnamon stick
¾ cup raisins
2 to 3 pinches sea salt
2 teaspoons vanilla extract
¼ cup kudzu
¼ cup purified water

For the dough:
⅔ cup organic whole wheat pastry flour
⅔ cup organic unbleached flour
1 pinch sea salt
2 ounces safflower oil
½ cup water

Optional garnish:
ground cinnamon

To make the filling:
1. In a large pan over medium heat, combine the apples, brown rice syrup, apple juice, cinnamon stick, raisins and salt. Bring to a boil and simmer for 20 minutes.
2. In a small bowl, dissolve the kudzu in water.
3. Add the vanilla extract and kudzu mixture to the pan and cook for 2 more minutes. Allow to cool and set aside.

To make the dough:
1. In a large bowl, combine the flours and sea salt.
2. In a small bowl, whisk together the oil and water and add to the flour mixture.
3. Stir gently by hand until the dough is uniform.
4. Using a rolling pin on a flat surface, roll dough into a rectangle about 8 x 12 inches, adding flour if necessary.

To assemble the strudel:
1. Preheat the oven to 350° F.
2. Place the apples lengthwise along the center of the dough. Starting on one of the long sides, roll the dough to form a log with the apples inside. Pinch the edges closed and place log on a baking pan lined with parchment paper.
3. Bake for 40 minutes. Remove from the oven and allow to cool. Slice into equal portions and garnish with ground cinnamon.

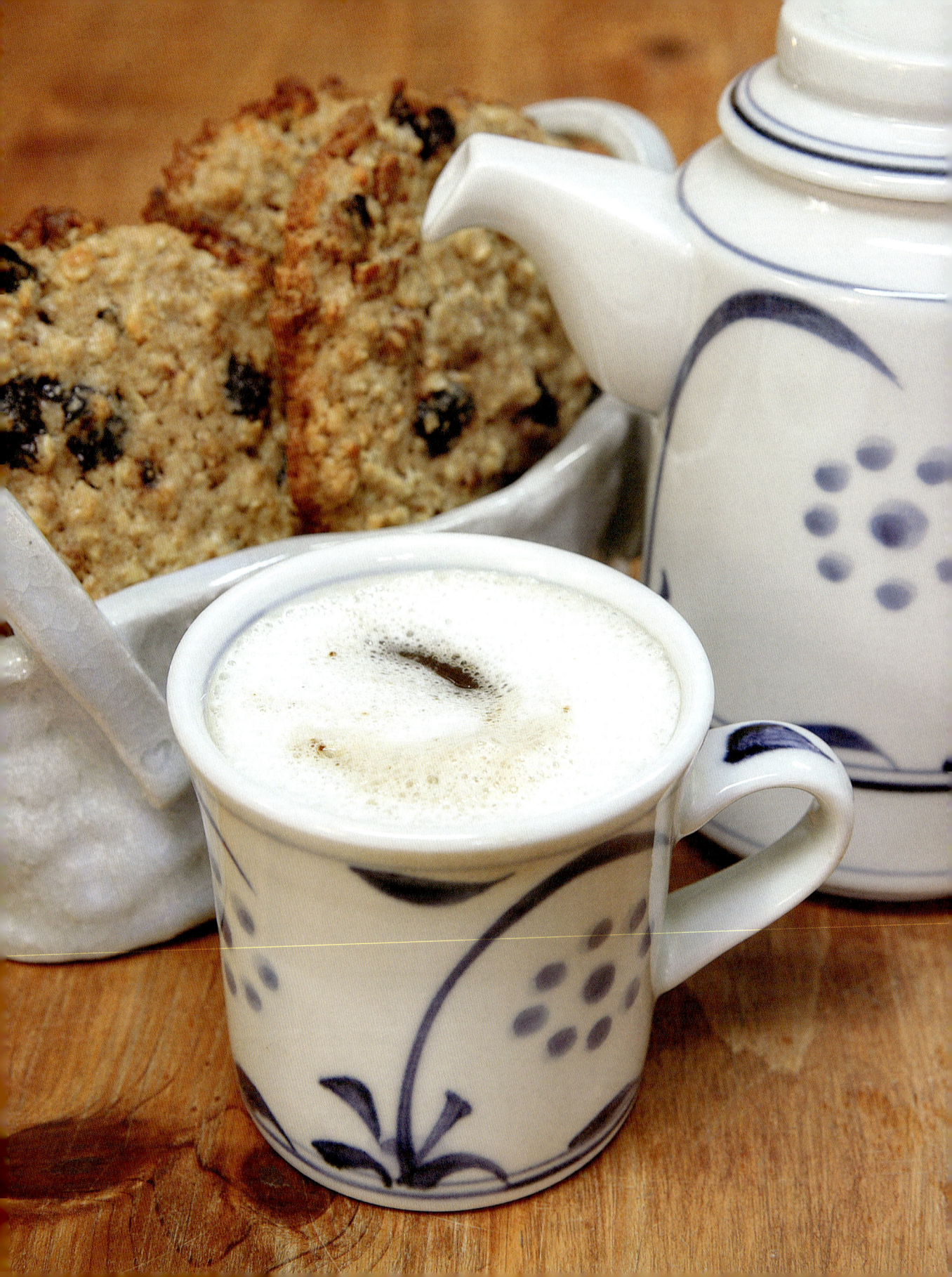

Oatmeal cherry kisses

Oatmeal cookie lovers shouldn't miss this one. We added cherries instead of raisins to give a kiss and a little love.

MAKES 12 COOKIES

For the cookies:
1 cup rolled oats
1 cup spelt flour
½ cup organic unbleached flour
½ tablespoon baking powder
¼ teaspoon sea salt
½ teaspoon coriander
1 cup chopped pecans
¾ cup dry cherries
½ cup brown rice syrup
¼ cup maple syrup
1 cup organic apple juice
¾ cup safflower oil
2 teaspoons vanilla extract

To make the cookies:
1. In a large bowl, combine the oats, flours, baking powder, sea salt, and coriander.
2. Add remaining ingredients and mix well to form a dough.
3. Refrigerate cookie dough for 2 hours.
4. Preheat the oven to 350° F.
5. Using a 2-ounce ice cream scoop, drop cookie dough about 2 inches apart onto a baking pan lined with parchment paper.
6. Bake for 20 minutes, or until golden brown.

Soy latte grain coffee

Once in a while, we make this hot drink treat so that we can still feel like a part of the coffee culture.

MAKES 2 SERVINGS

For the coffee:
4 tablespoons grain coffee*
2 cups soy milk (unsweetened)

*see glossary entry on page 100

To make the coffee:
1. In a small saucepan over low-medium heat, combine the grain coffee and the soy milk.
2. Gently simmer the coffee until it is hot and grain coffee has dissolved, but do not boil.
3. Pour into a French press until the press is half full. Pump repeatedly until the coffee reaches the desired level of foam.
4. Pour into a cup. Drink while hot.

BASIC ESSENTIALS

Cookie cutters
Baking pan, 12- x 17-inch
Muffin pan
Skillet, 10-inch
Sauté pan, 12-inch
Wok
Saucepan, 3-quart
Saucepan, 5-quart
Ramekins, shallow 4-inch

Mixing bowls
Rolling pin
Pickle press*
Pastry brush
Peeler
Corer
Ice cream scoop, 2-ounce
Melon ball scoop
Vegetable slicer (mandoline)
Fiber scrub brush
Parchment paper

Blender
Food processor

*Pickle pressers are available from Asian markets or health food markets that carry macrobiotic foods. If you don't have a press you can use a bowl and place a plate inside the bowl to press the fruit or vegetables.

METRIC CONVERSION

Temperature
Fahrenheit to Celsius

F	C
200 – 205	95
229 – 225	105
245 – 250	120
275	135
300 – 305	150
325 – 330	165
345 – 350	175
370 – 375	190
400 – 405	205
425 – 430	220
445 – 450	230
470 – 475	245
500	260

Liquid And Dry Measures

US	Metric
¼ teaspoon	1.25 milliliters
½ teaspoon	2.5 milliliters
1 teaspoon	5 milliliters
1 tablespoon	15 milliliters
¼ cup	60 milliliters
⅓ cup	80 milliliters
1 cup	240 milliliters
1 pint (2 cups)	480 milliliters
1 quart (4 cups)	960 milliliters
1 gallon (4 quarts)	3.84 liters
1 ounce (ounce)	28 grams
1 pound (16 ounces)	454 grams
2.2 pounds	1 kilogram

Length Measures

US	Metric
⅛ inch	3 millimeters
¼ inch	6 millimeters
½ inch	12 millimeters
1 inch	2.5 centimeters

INDEX

A
agar: 98
    Strawberry Cupcakes, 21
alfalfa sprouts: 98
    Shredded Daikon Salad
        with Pink Peppercorns, 65
almond(s): 98
    Country Whole Barley with Fava Beans, 18
    Apricot Linzer, 25
Apple Cinnamon Strudel, 87
Apricot Linzer, 25
arame: 98
    Arame Poppyseed Rolls, 48
Autumn recipe section, 58

B
barbecue:
    Grilled Nectarines with Lemon
        and Maple Glaze, 39
barley: 98, 99
    Country Whole Barley with Fava Beans, 18
basil: 100, 103
    Dulse and Cucumber with Basil, 36
    Sweet Corn Chowder with Basil Oil, 45
    Melon and Thai Basil Pickles
        with Lemongrass, 52
bean(s): 99, 100
    Country Whole Barley with Fava Beans, 18
    Butternut Squash and Kidney Bean Potage, 61
beet(s):
    Stuffed Shiitake Mushrooms
        with Millet and Kudzu Beet Sauce, 51
    Shredded Daikon Salad
        with Pink Peppercorns, 65
berries:
    Strawberry Cupcakes, 23
    Mini Blueberry Scones, 57
black sesame seed(s): 98
    Scrambled Tofu Florentine
        with Hollandaise Sauce, 35
    Black Sesame Dumplings
        with Warm Coconut Soup, 71

blueberries:
    Mini Blueberry Scones, 57
Braised Whole Burdock, 84
Breaded Rice Balls with Lotus Seeds, 64
brown rice: 98
    Country Whole Barley with Fava Beans, 18
    Breaded Rice Balls with Lotus Seeds, 64
    Genmaicha, 73
    Buckwheat and Brown Rice, 79
buckwheat: 98
    Buckwheat and Brown Rice, 79
Burdock: 98
    Braised Whole Burdock, 84
butternut: 98
    Butternut Squash and Kidney Bean Potage, 61

C
cabbage:
    Pressed Wakame and Napa Cabbage Rolls, 18
    Vegetable Pancakes with Tofu Sour Cream, 31
    Savoy Cabbage
        with Walnut and Carrot Sauce, 83
cantaloupe:
    Honeydew Melon Soup, 29
    Melon and Thai Basil Pickles
        with Lemongrass, 52
Caper(s): 99
    Tempeh Crab Cakes with Caper Sauce, 21
carrot(s):
    Carrot and Garbanzo Soup
        with Lotus Root and Dill, 15
    Vegetable Pancakes with Tofu Sour Cream, 31
    Scrambled Tofu Florentine
        with Hollandaise Sauce, 35
    Arame Poppyseed Rolls, 48
    Stuffed Shiitake Mushrooms
        with Millet and Kudzu Beet Sauce, 51
    Butternut Squash and Kidney Bean Potage, 61
    Root Vegetable Pot Pie, 63
    Breaded Rice Balls with Lotus Seeds, 64
    Lotus Root Pickles, 67

Seitan Bourguignon, 79
　　　Savoy Cabbage
　　　　with Walnut and Carrot Sauce, 83
cauliflower:
　　　Leek and Cauliflower Filo Wrap
　　　　with Mint Sauce, 17
celery:
　　　Carrot and Garbanzo Soup
　　　　with Lotus Root and Dill, 15
　　　Sweet Corn Chowder with Basil Oil, 45
　　　Stuffed Shiitake Mushrooms
　　　　with Millet and Kudzu Beet Sauce, 51
　　　Breaded Rice Balls with Lotus Seeds, 64
chamomile: 99
　　　Green Tea with Chamomile, 25
cherries:
　　　Oatmeal Cherry Kisses, 89
chickpeas (garbanzo beans): 100
　　　Carrot and Garbanzo Soup
　　　　with Lotus Root and Dill, 15
chocolate: 100
　　　Pistachio Chocolate Mouse, 55
chowder:
　　　Sweet Corn Chowder with Basil Oil, 45
cilantro: 99
　　　Leek and Cauliflower Filo Wrap
　　　　with Mint Sauce, 17
cinnamon:
　　　Apple Cinnamon Strudel, 87
coconut: 99
　　　Apricot Linzer, 25
　　　Black Sesame Dumplings
　　　　with Warm Coconut Soup, 71
coffee, grain: 100
　　　Soy Latte Grain Coffee, 89
cookies:
　　　Apricot Linzer, 25
　　　Hazelnut Baci, 41
　　　Walnut Cookies, 73
　　　Oatmeal Cherry Kisses, 89

corn:
　　　Cool Roasted Corn Tea, 41
　　　Sweet Corn Chowder with Basil Oil, 45
cucumber:
　　　Dulse and Cucumber with Basil, 36
cupcakes:
　　　Strawberry Cupcakes, 23
curry powder: 104
　　　Butternut Squash and Kidney Bean Potage, 61

D
daikon: 99
　　　Shredded Daikon Salad
　　　　with Pink Peppercorns, 65
dashi:
　　　Carrot and Garbanzo Soup
　　　　with Lotus Root and Dill, 15
　　　Kombu Dashi, 15
　　　Sweet Corn Chowder with Basil Oil, 45
　　　Root Vegetable Pot Pie, 63
　　　French Onion Soup with Crispy Mochi, 77
　　　Seitan Bourguignon, 79
　　　Savoy Cabbage
　　　　with Walnut and Carrot Sauce, 83
　　　Braised Whole Burdock, 84
desserts:
　　　Strawberry Cupcakes, 23
　　　Apricot Linzer, 25
　　　Grilled Nectarines
　　　　with Lemon and Maple Glaze, 39
　　　Hazelnut Baci, 41
　　　Pistachio Chocolate Mousse, 55
　　　Mini Blueberry Scones, 57
　　　Black Sesame Dumplings
　　　　with Warm Coconut Soup, 71
　　　Walnut Cookies, 73
　　　Apple Cinnamon Strudel, 87
　　　Oatmeal Cherry Kisses, 89
dill:
　　　Carrot and Garbanzo Soup
　　　　with Lotus Root and Dill, 15

dressings:
    for Inca Quinoa
        and Mustard Greens Salad, 32
    for Shredded Daikon Salad, 65
    Ginger Dressing, for Persimmon
        and Watercress with Asian Pear, 68
dulse: 99
    Dulse and Cucumber with Basil, 36
dumplings:
    Black Sesame Dumplings
        with Warm Coconut Soup, 71

E
edamame: 99
    Mihama Hijiki with Edamame
        and Roasted Pumpkin Seeds, 67
equipment list, 90

F
fava beans: 99
    Country Whole Barley with Fava Beans, 18
filberts (hazelnuts): 100
    Hazelnut Baci, 41
filo dough: 99
    Leek and Cauliflower Filo Wrap
        with Mint Sauce, 17
flour, (see oat flour, spelt flour, and pastry flour)
    23, 25, 31, 32, 41, 48, 57, 63, 64, 71, 73, 77,
    79, 87, 89, 99, 101, 103, 104
flowers: 99
    Green Tea with Chamomile, 25
    Kukicha with Rose Hips and Petals, 57
French Onion Soup with Crispy Mochi, 77
frosting:
    for Strawberry Cupcakes, 23

G
garbanzo beans: 100
    Carrot and Garbanzo Soup
        with Lotus Root and Dill, 15
Genmaicha, 73, 100

ginger:
    Leek and Cauliflower Filo Wrap
        with Mint Sauce, 17
    Ginger Dressing, for Persimmon
        and Watercress with Asian Pear, 68
glossary, 98
grains:
    Country Whole Barley with Fava Beans, 18
    Inca Quinoa and Mustard Greens Salad, 32
    Cool Roasted Corn Tea, 41
    Stuffed Shiitake Mushrooms
        with Millet and Kudzu Beet Sauce, 51
    Breaded Rice Balls with Lotus Seeds, 64
    Genmaicha, 73
    Buckwheat and Brown Rice, 79
Green Tea with Chamomile, 25
greens: 99, 101
    Sautéed Pea Sprouts, 21
    Inca Quinoa and Mustard Greens Salad, 32
    Red Radish and Green Top Pickles, 80
Grilled Nectarines
    with Lemon and Maple Glaze, 39

H
hazelnut(s): 100
    Hazelnut Baci, 41
hijiki: 100
    Mihama Hijiki with Edamame
        and Roasted Pumpkin Seeds, 67
Hollandaise Sauce,
    Scrambled Tofu Florentine with, 35
Honeydew Melon Soup, 29

I
Inca Quinoa and Mustard Greens Salad, 32

J
jinenjo: 100
    Root Vegetable Pot Pie, 63

K
kale: 100
  Scrambled Tofu Florentine
    with Hollandaise Sauce, 35
kamut: 100
  Kamut Spaghetti with Pine Nuts
    and Sun Dried Tomatoes, 47
kelp (as kombu), 100
kidney beans: 100
  Butternut Squash and Kidney Bean Potage, 61
kombu: 100
  Carrot and Garbanzo Soup
    with Lotus Root and Dill, 15
  Kombu Dashi, 15
  Sweet Corn Chowder with Basil Oil, 45
  Simmered Turnips, 47
  Butternut Squash and Kidney Bean Potage, 61
  Root Vegetable Pot Pie, 63
  French Onion Soup with Crispy Mochi, 77
  Crispy Kombu Chips, 80
  Savoy Cabbage
    with Walnut and Carrot Sauce, 83
  Braised Whole Burdock, 84
kudzu: 100
  Vegetable Pancakes with Tofu Sour Cream, 31
  Kudzu Beet Sauce, 51
  Root Vegetable Pot Pie, 63
  Apple Cinnamon Strudel, 87
Kukicha: 101
  Kukicha with Rose Hips and Petals, 57

L
Late Summer recipe section, 42
Leek and Cauliflower Filo Wrap
    with Mint Sauce, 17
lemon(s):
  Lemon and Maple Glaze,
    Grilled Nectarines with, 39
lemongrass: 101
  Melon and Thai Basil Pickles
    with Lemongrass, 52

Lotus: 101
  Carrot and Garbanzo Soup
    with Lotus Root and Dill, 15
  Breaded Rice Balls with Lotus Seeds, 64
  Lotus Root Pickles, 67

M
maple syrup (and granulated): 101
  Strawberry Cupcakes, 23
  Apricot Linzer, 25
  Zucchini Muffins, 32
  Maple Glaze, Grilled Nectarines
    with Lemon and, 39
  Hazelnut Baci, 41
  Pistachio Chocolate Mousse, 55
  Mini Blueberry Scones, 57
  Walnut Cookies, 73
  Oatmeal Cherry Kisses, 89
melon(s):
  Honeydew Melon Soup, 29
  Melon and Thai Basil Pickles
    with Lemongrass, 52
Mihama Hijiki with Edamame
    and Roasted Pumpkin Seeds, 67
millet: 101
  Stuffed Shiitake Mushrooms
    with Millet and Kudzu Beet Sauce, 51
mint:
  Mint Sauce, Leek and Cauliflower
    Filo Wrap with, 17
  Honeydew Melon Soup, 29
miso, white/country barley: 99, 104
  Carrot and Garbanzo Soup
    with Lotus Root and Dill, 15
  Sweet Corn Chowder with Basil Oil, 45
  Butternut Squash
    and Kidney Bean Potage, 61
  Persimmon and Watercress
    with Asian Pear, 68
  French Onion Soup with Crispy Mochi, 77
mochi: 101
  French Onion Soup with Crispy Mochi, 77

mousse:
    Pistachio Chocolate Mousse, 55
muffins:
    Zucchini Muffins, 32
mushrooms:
    Stuffed Shiitake Mushrooms
        with Millet and Kudzu Beet Sauce, 51
mustard greens: 101
    Inca Quinoa and Mustard Greens Salad, 32

N
Napa cabbage:
    Pressed Wakame and Napa Cabbage Rolls, 18
nectarines:
    Grilled Nectarines
        with Lemon and Maple Glaze, 39
nuts: 100, 102, 104
    Apricot Linzer, 25
    Hazelnut Baci, 41
    Kamut Spaghetti with Pine Nuts
        and Sun Dried Tomatoes, 47
    Pistachio Chocolate Mousse, 55
    Walnut Cookies, 73

O
oat(s)/oat flour: 101, 102
    Srawberry Cupcakes, 23
    Hazelnut Baci, 41
    Oatmeal Cherry Kisses, 89
Oatmeal Cherry Kisses, 89
Onion Soup, French, with Crispy Mochi, 77
onions, pearl: 102
    Seitan Bourguignon, 79

P
pancakes:
    Vegetable Pancakes with Tofu Sour Cream, 31
parsnips:
    Root Vegetable Pot Pie, 63
pasta:
    Kamut Spaghetti with Pine Nuts
        and Sun Dried Tomatoes, 47
pastry flour: 101
    Apricot Linzer, 25
    Hazelnut Baci, 41
    Arame Poppyseed Rolls, 48
    Mini Blueberry Scones, 57
    Root Vegetable Pot Pie, 63
    Walnut Cookies, 73
    Apple Cinnamon Strudel, 87
patties:
    Tempeh Crab Cakes with Caper Sauce, 21
pea sprouts: 102
    Sautéed Pea Sprouts, 21
pear:
    Persimmon and Watercress with Asian Pear, 68
peas, sugar snap:
    Carrot and Garbanzo Soup
        with Lotus Root and Dill, 15
pecans: 102
    Oatmeal Cherry Kisses, 89
peppercorns, pink: 102
    Shredded Daikon Salad
        with Pink Peppercorns, 65
peppers, green/red:
    Tempeh Crab Cakes with Caper Sauce, 21
Persimmon and Watercress with Asian Pear, 68
pickle(s): 90
    Pressed Wakame and Napa Cabbage Rolls, 18
    Dulse and Cucumber with Basil, 36
    Melon and Thai Basil Pickles
        with Lemongrass, 52
    Lotus Root Pickles, 67
    Red Radish and Green Top Pickles, 80
pie(s):
    Arame Poppyseed Rolls, 48
    Root Vegetable Pot Pie, 63
pine nuts: 102
    Kamut Spaghetti with Pine Nuts
        and Sun Dried Tomatoes, 47
pistachio(s): 100
    Pistachio Chocolate Mousse, 55
poppyseed(s): 102
    Arame Poppyseed Rolls, 48

Pressed Wakame and Napa Cabbage Rolls, 18
puff pastry:
    Root Vegetable Pot Pie, 63
pumpkin seeds: 102
    Mihama Hijiki with Edamame
        and Roasted Pumpkin Seeds, 67

Q

quinoa, red: 102
    Inca Quinoa and Mustard Greens Salad, 32

R

radish(es), red: 102
    Red Radish and Green Top Pickles, 80
rice, brown: 98
    Country Whole Barley with Fava Beans, 18
    Breaded Rice Balls with Lotus Seeds, 64
    Genmaicha, 73
    Buckwheat and Brown Rice, 79
Root Vegetable Pot Pie, 63
rose, hips and petals: 102
    Kukicha with Rose Hips and Petals, 57
Ryokucha: 103
    Green Tea with Chamomile, 25

S

saffron: 103
    Lotus Root Pickles, 67
salads:
    Pressed Wakame and Napa Cabbage Rolls, 18
    Sautéed Pea Sprouts, 21
    Inca Quinoa and Mustard Greens Salad, 32
    Dulse and Cucumber with Basil, 36
    Melon and Thai Basil Pickles
        with Lemongrass, 52
    Shredded Daikon Salad
        with Pink Peppercorns, 65
    Lotus Root Pickles, 67
    Persimmon and Watercress with Asian Pear, 68
    Red Radish and Green Top Pickles, 80
Savoy Cabbage with Walnut and Carrot Sauce, 83

scallion(s):
    Vegetable Pancakes with Tofu Sour Cream, 31
    Breaded Rice Balls with Lotus Seeds, 64
    Lotus Root Pickles, 67
scones:
    Mini Blueberry Scones, 57
Scrambled Tofu Florentine
    with Hollandaise Sauce, 35
sea vegetable(s): 98, 99, 100, 104
    Kombu Dashi, 15
    Pressed Wakame and Napa Cabbage Rolls, 18
    Dulse and Cucumber with Basil, 36
    Arame Poppyseed Rolls, 48
    Mihama Hijiki with Edamame
        and Roasted Pumpkin Seeds, 67
    Crispy Kombu Chips, 80
seitan: 103
    Seitan Bourguignon, 79
sesame, [see black sesame seed(s)]
shiitake: 103
    Stuffed Shiitake Mushrooms
        with Millet and Kudzu Beet Sauce, 51
    Root Vegetable Pot Pie, 63
shiso: 103
    Shredded Daikon Salad
        with Pink Peppercorns, 65
Shredded Daikon Salad
    with Pink Peppercorns, 65
Simmered Turnips, 47
soup(s):
    Carrot and Garbanzo Soup
        with Lotus Root and Dill, 15
    Kombu Dashi, 15
    Honeydew Melon Soup, 29
    Sweet Corn Chowder with Basil Oil, 45
    Butternut Squash and Kidney Bean Potage, 61
    Black Sesame Dumplings
        with Warm Coconut Soup, 71
    French Onion Soup with Crispy Mochi, 77
soy: 99, 103, 104
    Mihama Hijiki with Edamame
        and Roasted Pumpkin Seeds, 67

Soy Latte Grain Coffee, 89
(also see edamame, tofu, tempeh, and miso)
spaghetti, kamut: 100
    Kamut Spaghetti with Pine Nuts
        and Sun Dried Tomatoes, 47
spelt flour: 103
    Strawberry Cupcakes, 23
    Zucchini Muffins, 32
    French Onion Soup with Crispy Mochi, 77
Spring recipe section, 12
sprouts, pea: 102
    Sautéed Pea Sprouts, 21
squash, butternut: 98
    Butternut Squash and Kidney Bean Potage, 61
Stuffed Shiitake Mushrooms
    with Millet and Kudzu Beet Sauce, 51
strawberries:
    Strawberry Cupcakes, 23
strudel:
    Apple Cinnamon Strudel, 87
sugar snap peas:
    Carrot and Garbanzo Soup
        with Lotus Root and Dill, 15
Summer:
    Summer Brunch recipe section, 26
    Late Summer recipe section, 42
Sweet Corn Chowder with Basil Oil, 45

T

tea: 100, 102, 103
    Green Tea with Chamomile, 25
    Cool Roasted Corn Tea, 41
    Kukicha with Rose Hips and Petals, 57
    Genmaicha, 73
Tempeh: 8, 103
    Tempeh Crab Cakes with Caper Sauce, 21
thai basil: 103
    Melon and Thai Basil Pickles
        with Lemongrass, 52
tofu: 103, 104
    Tempeh Crab Cakes with Caper Sauce, 21
    Strawberry Cupcakes, 23

Tofu Sour Cream, Vegetable Pancakes with, 31
Scrambled Tofu Florentine
    with Hollandaise Sauce, 35
Pistachio Chocolate Mousse, 55
Mini Blueberry Scones, 57
Walnut Cookies, 73
tomato(es):
    Scrambled Tofu Florentine
        with Hollandaise Sauce, 35
    Kamut Spaghetti with Pine Nuts
        and Sun Dried Tomatoes, 47
turnip(s): 104
    Simmered Turnips, 47
twig tea, (as Kukicha): 100
    Kukicha with Rose Hips and Petals, 57

V

Vegenaise: 104
    Tempeh Crab Cakes with Caper Sauce, 21
    Scrambled Tofu Florentine
        with Hollandaise Sauce, 35
Vegetable Pancakes with Tofu Sour Cream, 31

W

wakame, 18, 104
    Pressed Wakame and Napa Cabbage Rolls, 18
walnut(s): 104
    Walnut Cookies, 73
    Walnut and Carrot Sauce,
        Savoy Cabbage with, 83
watercress:
    Persimmon and Watercress with Asian Pear, 68
Winter recipe section, 74

Y

yogurt, soy: 103
    Honeydew Melon Soup, 29

Z

Zucchini Muffins, 32

GLOSSARY

Agar agar
A sea vegetable that comes in bar or flake form. Used for making gelatins and aspics.

Alfalfa sprouts
Germinated from alfalfa seeds and harvested as a nutritious food. A popular addition to salads and sandwiches, providing crispness as an ingredient.

Almonds
Fruit kernels of the almond tree. They keep best when purchased in their brown skins, which protect their freshness and flavor.

Arame
A sea vegetable in the form of many long brown or black strands. Mildly flavored, it is usually used as a side dish.

Baking powder
A leavening agent made of baking soda, cream of tartar, and either cornstarch or arrowroot. It releases carbon dioxide upon contact with liquid, creating air pockets which create a light texture in baked goods.

Baking soda
A leavening agent used in baking. It releases carbon dioxide upon contact with liquid, creating air pockets which create a light texture in baked goods.

Barley
One of the most widely grown grains after wheat and corn. Barley and products made from it are useful in a variety of ways, and tend to be healthier than products made from wheat or corn.

Black sesame paste
A paste made from black sesame seeds. Sesame seeds are high in oil content, and have excellent antioxidant properties.

Brown rice
Whole, unpolished rice, containing an ideal balance of minerals, protein and carbohydrates.

Brown rice syrup
A sweetener made from fermented brown rice, that provides a steady source of energy after consumption for several hours.

Brown rice vinegar
A mild vinegar made by fermenting brown rice.

Buckwheat
A grain used similarly to wheat, although it is not actually related to common strains of wheat. Usually associated with an earthy, full taste.

Burdock root
A long, thick root vegetable used in various soups and salads. It has an earthy flavor, similar to an artichoke.

Butternut squash
A winter squash with an abundance of solid flesh. Creamy-textured when cooked, the butternut squash is particularly delectable in various soups.

Capers
Small berries with a strong, pungent flavor. Used for flavoring, they are often packed in brine, making them taste very salty.

Caraway seeds
A common spice, often used in breads, cheeses, and curries.

Chamomile flowers
An herb that has been cultivated since ancient times, most often valued for its sweet scent and for its calming medicinal properties.

Cilantro
Also known as Chinese parsley, cilantro has a very distinct flavor and is commonly used in Mexican and Asian dishes.

Coconut powder
Made from the dried, ground flesh of a mature coconut, it can come either sweetened or unsweetened. For the recipes in this book, make sure to use unsweetened varieties.

Coriander
A valuable spice, often used as a scent in various industries. In food preparation, it is often used for flavoring vegetables, pickles and curries.

Country barley miso
A variety of miso (a thick, salty paste made from soybeans, sea salt and fermented grains) that is often thought to be the most medicinal and made from both soybeans and barley.

Curry powder
A blend of spices formulated in East India that usually includes turmeric. The spiciness of curry powder varies widely depending on the exact type and amount of the ingredients.

Daikon
A Japanese white radish, used in many dishes. It is said to have properties that help dissolve deposits of fat and mucus in the body.

Dulse
A reddish seaweed that can be eaten "wet" or "dry." In wet form (straight out of the package) it can be very salty, and in dry form (after baking or toasting) it can add a pleasing crunch to salads or wherever desired.

Edamame
Green soybeans, usually served still in the pod. They may be eaten raw or after roasting, boiling, or baking.

Fava beans
Very hardy beans that are usually quite large and come in flat, light-green pods about eight inches long.

Filo dough
An eastern-European pastry dough made by using many paper-thin sheets to form a light, crumbly offering. Available in white or whole wheat flour.

Garbanzo beans
Also known as chickpeas, these fleshy beans are the main ingredient in hummus.

Genmaicha
A tea made of roasted leaves and brown rice, used for making tea.

Grain coffee
A coffee substitute made of roasted grains, beans and roots. It contains no caffeine. In macrobiotics, it is considered an occasional beverage.

Grain mustard
Condiment containing whole mustard seeds.

Grain-sweetened chocolate chips
Sweetened with grain syrup instead of sugar.

Green nori flakes
Flakes of pressed green nori sea vegetable (different than the more common black nori used in sushi rolls) that can be used as a condiment on many dishes.

Ground pistachio
A powder made from the flavorful pistachio nut.

Hazelnuts
Also known as filberts, these are nuts shaped like large chickpeas. They have a very bitter outer skin that must be removed before eating.

Herbs de Provence
A collection of herbs, usually mixed together and referred to by this name. Herbs de Provence usually contains marjoram, savory, fennel, basil, thyme and lavender.

Hijiki
A strong, thick sea vegetable known for its richness in calcium, hijiki is delicious when combined with strong seasonings.

Jinenjo potatoes
Japanese mountain yams.

Kale
A relative of cabbage and collard greens, kale is a delicious vegetable that is best if steamed, blanched or sautéed. High in calcium and magnesium.

Kamut spaghetti
Spaghetti made from kamut, a variety of Egyptian wheat. Available through health and natural food stores.

Kidney beans
Dark red, kidney-shaped beans, among the most popular beans in the United States.

Kombu
A sea vegetable, often called the "king of seaweed." Although related to kelp, and notable for its mild, salty flavor, kombu is actually quite soft and easily incorporated into many dishes in a variety of ways.

Kudzu (kuzu)
A wild plant root used to make a white starch. Also known as kudzu root.

Kukicha
Also known as "twig tea," kukicha is made from the twigs and leaves of Japanese twig bushes.

Lemongrass
A lemon-scented grass often used as a flavoring or garnish in Southeast Asian dishes.

Lotus root
A hollow-chambered root much like a potato, lotus root is used in several vegetable dishes and home remedies. It is also the root of the lotus lily, which is a beautiful addition to any dinner table.

Lotus seeds
Seeds from the lotus plant, usually purchased shelled and dried. They must be soaked extensively before adding to the intended dish.

Maple syrup
The boiled-down sap of the sugar maple tree which can be used as a natural flavoring and sweetener. Do not confuse this with "maple-flavored" syrup, which is usually mostly sugar or corn syrup.

Maple sugar
A powdered form of maple syrup. Used as a sweetener either baked into desserts or sprinkled on top of them.

Millet
A small, round yellow grain, often used in place of buckwheat, rice or quinoa, that is rich in B-vitamins. Historically, millet is a staple in West Indian bread-making.

Mirin
A cooking wine with a powerful flavor made from sweet brown rice. It is often used to flavor fish.

Mochi
A rice cake or dumpling made from cooked, pounded sweet rice.

Mustard greens
A rich, darkly-colored green that tastes strongly of mustard. A staple of East Indian dishes.

Nayonnaise
See "Vegenaise" listing.

Oat flour
Flour made from grinding oat groats to a fine consistency. This may be done on your own by grinding rolled oats in a blender. It is very low in gluten, so use with a gluten-containing flour to help your bread rise.

Paprika
A spice made from powdered sweet red peppers. Traditionally used as a flavoring and coloring for rices, stews and soups.

Pastry flour
Special flour that is particularly high in gluten (wheat protein) and is more suitable for light, fine pastries. Available in white or whole wheat.

Pea sprouts
A delicate, sweet sprout used to add moisture and texture to sandwiches and salads.

Pearl onions
Small, round, white onions with a slightly sweet taste. Make sure they have a firm, clear skin without bruises, and store in a woven bag away from fluorescent lighting.

Pecans
A popular nut with a rich, buttery flavor. Used frequently in desserts, but can also make a delicious addition to some savory meals.

Pine nuts
An edible seed found inside pine cones. They have a soft texture and sweet flavor.

Pink peppercorns
The dried pink or red berries from the Brazilian pepper plant, a distant relation of the more common black pepper plant.

Poppyseeds
Small black seeds from the poppy plant, used to give a faint shift in taste, or for decoration.

Powdered rice syrup
A powder made from rice syrup, used as a sweetener or decoration for desserts.

Pumpkin seeds
Traditionally served as a snack in the autumn, roasted pumpkin seeds make an excellent addition to salads or vegetable dishes.

Red quinoa
An heirloom variety of quinoa, a grain with a particularly high protein content and complete set of amino acids. Rare among grains, quinoa also contains no gluten.

Red radishes
A firm, crispy vegetable that can be eaten raw or lightly cooked. The greens are also edible and can add a peppery taste to a salad or vegetable dish.

Rice milk
A grain milk made from brown or white rice. It contains more carbohydrates than cow's milk.

Rice syrup
A sweetener made by fermenting brown or white rice.

Rice vinegar
Rice vinegar made from brown or white rice. Has a lower acid content than most other vinegars, and is lighter in taste.

Rolled oats
Oats that have been processed by being rolled flat to have the thick outer husks removed. There are types of rolled oats that differ based on the size of the oat flakes and on whether they have been baked or pressure-cooked after rolling.

Rose hips and petals
The fruit and petals of the rose plant. High in vitamin C, rose hips and petals are often used to make teas.

Ryokucha
Leaves used to make Japanese green tea.

Safflower oil
Great for cooking, baking or as a salad oil.

Saffron
Good for the digestion, this bright red spice is commonly used as a flavoring or as an element in red dye.

Sea salt
Salt obtained from the ocean and either sun- or kiln-baked. Unlike refined table salt, it is high in trace minerals and contains no chemicals, sugar or other additives.

Seitan
Wheat protein cooked and kneaded into a meat substitute.

Shiitake mushrooms
Japanese mushrooms with a large cap with a meaty, smoky taste and chewy texture (even after cooking).

Shiso leaves
Also known as the beefsteak plant, shiso is a minty herb with large leaves used for flavoring. It is recognized for its anti-inflammatory properties.

Soy margarine
A high-protein butter substitute made from soy beans. Avoid brands containing hydrogenated oils.

Soy milk
The rich, creamy milk of whole soybeans. Usually sold as "soy beverage" or "soy drink", it is an excellent dairy substitute and is high in B-vitamins and protein.

Soy sauce
A flavoring made by aging soybeans, wheat, water and sea salt. Avoid brands with added alcohol and preservatives.

Soy yogurt
A yogurt made from soy milk. Available in sweetened or plain unsweetened varieties. Delicious!

Spelt flour
Made from a non-hybridized wheat, it works well as a bread flour and is very high in protein. It is a good substitute for people who are allergic to wheat. Available in refined white and whole grain varieties.

Sweet rice flour
Flour made from ground rice, either white or brown.

Tempeh
A high-protein food made from cultured soybeans (often with grain products added). Excellent as a meat substitute. Less processed than tofu.

Thai basil
A basil relative with smaller leaves and a stronger taste.

Tofu
Soybean curd made from soybeans and nigari (magnesium chloride) or calcium chloride. Tofu is very versatile. It can be fried, baked, added raw to soups and salads, or puréed and used as a dairy substitute.

Turmeric powder
A dark yellow spice from India, similar to ginger, and a major ingredient in Indian curries.

Turnips
A round, firm root vegetable related to rutabagas. When smaller, they are delicate and have a slightly sweet flavor, but as they age their taste becomes stronger and the flesh more woody.

Unbleached white flour
Popular due to its versatility, unbleached white flour can be used for breads, pastries, cookies and cakes. To enhance its nutritional quality, substitute part of the white flour with whole wheat flour.

Vanilla bean
The seed pod of the vanilla plant. When the bean or seeds are used instead of prepared vanilla extract, stronger flavors can be released into the food.

Vanilla extract
A smoky, smooth flavoring made by extracting the essence from vanilla beans. Available preserved with or without alcohol.

Vegenaise
An egg and dairy-free mayonnaise substitute. Follow Your Heart-brand Vegenaise is thicker and creamier than the lighter Nayonnaise brand.

Wakame
Commonly found in miso soup, wakame is one of the sweetest of the sea vegetables, and one of the easiest to include in meals of all types.

Walnuts
A thick, heavy nut with a woody shell, high in oils and omega-3 fatty acids.

White miso
A variety of miso (a thick, salty paste made from soybeans, sea salt and fermented grains) that uses white rice as an essential ingredient.

White wine vinegar
Vinegar made by oxidizing white wine.

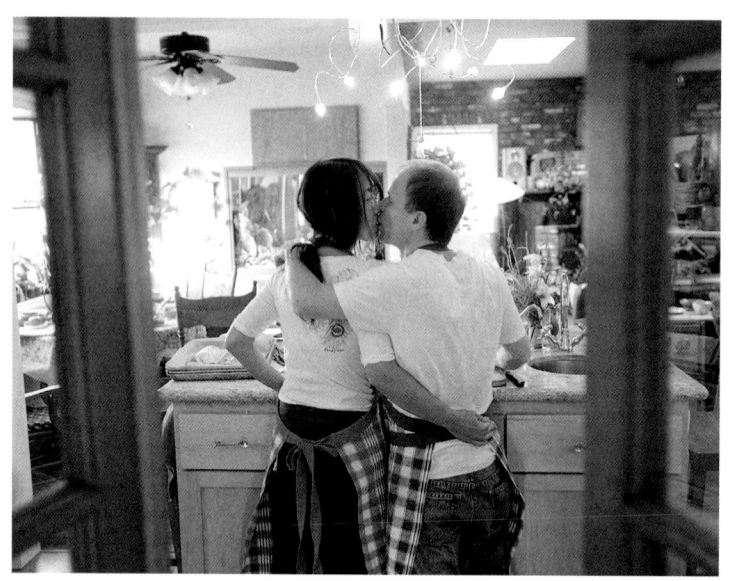